食 物 过 敏

——中西医结合疗法的探究

Food Allergies: Traditional Chinese Medicine, Western Science, and the Search for a Cure

原著　亨利·埃尔利希（Henry Ehrlich）

译者　郭先英　张加民　周义斌　骆世平

U0380357

东南大学出版社
SOUTHEAST UNIVERSITY PRESS

·南京·

内容提要

本书以李秀敏博士的研究为专业背景,以动物实验模型的建立为基础,分析了食物过敏诱发疾病的机制,通过量化指标详细介绍了中药及中西医结合方法治疗食物过敏引发的疾病的可能性及作用机制以及中药组方的疗效,为食物过敏性疾病的有效、规范治疗开辟了新路径。本书实验步骤科学、合理,数据真实、有效,结果可验证,为弘扬中医药文化提供了新的思路。

本书可供从事过敏性疾病研究及诊疗的相关人员使用,也可供中医药专业人士、在校学生参考使用。

图书在版编目(CIP)数据

食物过敏:中西医结合疗法的探究 /(美)亨利·埃尔利希(Henry Ehrlich)著;郭先英等译. —南京:东南大学出版社,2020.8

书名原文:Food Allergies:Traditional Chinese Medicine, Western Science, and the Search for a Cure

ISBN 978-7-5641-9028-6

Ⅰ.①食… Ⅱ.①亨… ②郭… Ⅲ.①食物过敏-中西医结合疗法-研究 Ⅳ.①R593.105

中国版本图书馆 CIP 数据核字(2020)第 135286 号

食物过敏:中西医结合疗法的探究

Shiwu Guomin:Zhongxiyi Jiehe Liaofa de Tanjiu

| 著　　者 | 亨利·埃尔利希 | 译　　者 | 郭先英 | 张加民 | 周义斌 | 骆世平 |

责任编辑　刘 坚　　　电　话　(025)83793329　QQ:635353748　电子邮件　liu-jian@seu.edu.cn

出版发行　东南大学出版社　　　　　　　　　出 版 人　江建中
地　　址　南京市四牌楼 2 号(210096)　　　邮　编　210096
销售电话　(025)83794561/83794174/83794121/83795801/83792174/83795802/57711295(传真)
网　　址　http://www.seupress.com　　　　　电子邮件　press@seupress.com

经　　销　全国各地新华书店　　　　　　　印　刷　虎彩印艺股份有限公司
开　　本　787 mm×1092 mm　1/16　　　印　张　12.25　字　数　350 千字
版　　次　2020 年 8 月第 1 版　　　　　印　次　2020 年 8 月第 1 次
书　　号　ISBN 978-7-5641-9028-6
定　　价　60.00 元

NOTES ON THE TEXT

Dr. Li thanks the National Institutes of Health (NIH) for supporting her basic and clinical research, and FARE (Food Allergy Research and Education—formerly Food-Allergy Initiative for supporting her work into clinical trials). She is also very grateful to funds directly established at Mount Sinai School of Medicine including the Winston Wolkoff Fund for Integrative Medicine for Allergies and Wellness (Contributors: Stephanie Winston Wolkoff and David Wolkoff, Barbara Winston, Ralph Lauren, Saks Inc.), Lisa Yu, the David L. Klein Jr. Foundation, Anna Sherbakova and Sergey Pichugov, Walter Alexander, Jonathan and Anne Garber, and Evan Fellman, Chris Burch Fund, Sean Parker Foundation, the Dugan family, and the Weissman family.

文本说明

李秀敏博士很感谢美国国立卫生研究院对其基础临床研究的支持,感谢食物过敏研究和教育协会,也就是原来的食物过敏协会支持她临床试验的工作。她也很感激直接设立在西奈山医学院的基金,包括资助针对过敏和健康的中西医结合医学研究的温斯顿·沃尔科夫基金(捐赠者:斯蒂芬妮·温斯顿·沃尔科夫和大卫·沃尔科夫、芭芭拉·温斯顿、拉尔夫·劳伦和萨克斯股份有限公司),余丽莎、小大卫·L.克莱因基金会、安娜·西切巴卡瓦和谢尔盖·皮丘戈夫、沃尔特·亚历山大、乔纳森和安妮·加伯以及埃文·费尔曼、克里斯·伯奇基金、西恩·帕克基金、杜根家族和维斯曼家族。

FOREWORD

John L. Lehr, CEO,
Food Allergy Research & Education

My first awareness of the seriousness of food allergies occurred when I met my step-nephew Zach several years before I became the Chief Executive Officer of Food Allergy Research & Education (FARE), the nation's leading food allergy research, education and advocacy organization. Zach, who is now 14, is allergic to milk, eggs, peanuts, tree nuts and shellfish. Soon after Zach became a part of my family, the daily challenges he had managing food allergies became apparent, as was the ever-present fear of anaphylaxis.

Since becoming CEO of FARE, I have met thousands of families struggling with the same issues and, tragically, a number of families who have lost their children to this insidious disease. Today, up to 15 million Americans are living with food allergies themselves and millions more when you include the accommodations made by their families and friends. While individuals take a number of precautions to successfully manage the disease, avoiding food allergens remains the only sure way to remain safe. Life-threatening reactions from accidental exposures are a reality, and the fact that a food allergy reaction sends someone to the emergency room every three minutes is a constant reminder of the need for a cure.

前　言

约翰·L.莱尔,
食物过敏研究和教育协会
首席执行官

我第一次意识到食物过敏的严重性是在我遇到我的继侄子扎克时,几年后,我成了食物过敏研究和教育协会(FARE)的首席执行官。FARE是美国食物过敏研究教育和倡议的领导组织。现年14岁的扎克对牛奶、鸡蛋、花生,坚果和贝类海鲜过敏。扎克成为我家庭的一员后不久,他在处理食物过敏问题上所面临的日常挑战和对过敏反应一直存在的恐惧就变得很明显。

在成为FARE的首席执行官之后,我遇到了成千上万跟食物过敏做斗争的家庭。可悲的是,很多家庭已经因为这种难治的疾病失去了他们的孩子。至今多达1500万的美国人患有食物过敏,如果你把和他们住在一起的家人和朋友包含在内的话,受到食物过敏影响的人能再多几百万。虽然人们采用各种各样的预防措施成功地控制这种疾病,但是避免接触到过敏原食物仍是保持安全的唯一可靠办法。由于意外接触过敏原而产生危及生命的过敏反应是真实存在的,并且,每三分钟就会有一个人因为过敏被送到急诊室,这样一个事实时刻提醒我们需要找到治愈的方法。

As the largest private funder of food allergy research in the world, FARE is committed to investing in science that will save lives. While food allergy research is still in the early stages, it is critical to explore innovative therapies and attract scientists from many fields and disciplines. Dr. Xiu-Min Li, a world-renowned scientist at Mount Sinai Medical Center, exemplifies those scientists.

In Henry Ehrlich's book *Food Allergies: Traditional Chinese Medicine, Western Science, and the Search for a Cure*, we follow Dr. Li's unique career as she investigates a potentially life-changing therapy for food allergies. The book reads like a medical thriller, as Dr. Li and her team explore an herbal formula developed from traditional Chinese medicine (TCM), and test this formula against the rigors of Western science. What ultimately follows is a deeper understanding of the complexities of human immunology, the interplay between TCM and Western medicine, and the dedication of the scientists who are working to solve this growing global health crisis. Although the author is a strict believer in laboratory and clinical research methods, and the importance of reporting research results in peer review journals, the patient stories Ehrlich presents at the end of the book offer anecdotal-but-compelling evidence of the promise of TCM as a viable therapeutic approach. Also in the thriller spirit, Ehrlich's book leads to a variety of exciting surprise endings including broader application of TCM in other diseases, explorations of possible avenues

作为世界上最大的食物过敏研究的私人资助的基金，FARE 致力于投资能够拯救生命的科学。尽管食物过敏研究现在还处于初级阶段，但探索创新疗法以及吸引来自许多不同领域和学科的科学家们极为重要。西奈山医学中心的李秀敏博士是世界著名的科学家，她为科学家们做了一个榜样。

在亨利·埃尔利希的《食物过敏——中西医结合疗法的探究》一书中，我们关注了李秀敏博士独特的事业，因为她在研究一种可能改变患者人生的食物过敏疗法。这本书读起来就像是一部医学惊险小说，李秀敏博士和她的团队探索从传统中医药（TCM）发展而来的中药方剂，并且用西方科学对这一配方进行了严格检验。最终，我们将对人类免疫学的复杂性、中医和西医之间的相互作用，以及致力于解决这一日益增长的全球健康危机的科学家们的奉献精神有更深入的理解。尽管作者严格相信实验室和临床研究方法，以及同行评论期刊中研究结果报告的重要性，埃尔利希在这本书的结尾所展示的病人的故事，为中医作为可行性治疗方法的前景提供了强有力的轶事证据。同时，在这种像"惊险小说"的精神中，埃尔利希的书引出了一系列激动人心的惊奇结果，包括中医在其他疾病治疗中的广泛应用，探索改变过敏症代际进程的可能途径，以及对中西医结合医学独特视角的展望。

to alter the inter-generational course of allergies, and prospects for a unique vision of integrative medicine.

Well-written and easy-to-follow, this book will serve as a great reference for those interested in food allergies, clinical research, and the different pathways that may lead to a cure.

这本书具有很高的学术价值,文笔流畅且通俗易懂。本书将为那些对食物过敏、临床研究和对不同食物过敏疗法感兴趣的学者们提供很好的参考。

INTRODUCTION

I first met Dr. Xiu-Min Li in 2010 when I visited her office at Mount Sinai Medical Center in New York on the recommendation of Dr. Paul Ehrlich, my cousin, coauthor and cofounder of a website devoted to pediatric allergies and asthma. Paul is not normally inclined toward alternative treatments. In fact, our project with Dr. Larry Chiaramonte, another pediatric allergist—the publication of *Asthma Allergies Children: A Parent's Guide* simultaneously with the launch of asthmaallergieschildren. com and related ventures—deals forthrightly with the guideline medicine they both practice, although we do have a section on alternatives, which mentions Chinese medicine. Paul said he had heard Dr. Li speak and, because she was working in one of the world's top allergy-research institutions, thought it was worth trying to get Dr. Li to contribute to our site.

As a lifelong reader of *The New York Times*, my first acquaintance with traditional Chinese medicine (TCM) came on July 26,1971, when the eminent columnist James Reston wrote about his emergency appendectomy while covering Henry Kissinger's visit to China. [①] The diagnosis and surgery were accomplished by a combination of TCM and Western medicine; however, his

---

① James Reston, The New York Times, July 26, 1971, http://www.acupuncture.com/testimonials/restonexp.htm.

序　言

我第一次见到李秀敏博士是在2010 年,那时我去她所在的纽约西奈山医学中心的办公室拜访她,是保罗·埃尔利希博士推荐我去的。保罗是我的堂兄,也是本书的合著者,我们共同创建了一个致力于儿童过敏和哮喘的网站。保罗一般不倾向于替代疗法。事实上,我们与另一位儿科过敏专家拉里·基亚拉蒙特博士合作出版《儿童过敏性哮喘:家长指南》的项目,以及同时推出的 asthmaallergieschildren. com 网站和相关公司,都直接涉及他们使用的参考药物,尽管我们确实有一个关于替代疗法的章节,其中提到了中药。保罗说他听过李秀敏博士的演讲,且李秀敏博士当时正在世界顶尖的过敏研究机构工作,所以他认为争取让李秀敏博士给我们的网站投稿是件值得努力的事情。

作为《纽约时报》的终身读者,我第一次接触中医是在 1971 年 7 月 26日。著名专栏作家詹姆斯·莱斯顿在报道亨利·基辛格访华时,谈到了自己的急性阑尾切除手术。他的诊断和外科手术采用了中西医结合的方法,而他巨大的术后痛苦是由针灸减轻的。41

considerable postoperative pain was relieved by acupuncture. Reading it again 41 years later, I was impressed by how vibrant TCM was both as an academic and a practical field back then. My own association with TCM was confined to the jars of dried vegetables on shelves in Chinatown stores. The idea of treating allergies with TCM sounded like rebuilding New York's infrastructure with plans for the Pyramids, the Parthenon, and St. Paul's Cathedral—not to mention any engineering marvels in China itself.

Dr. Li's office is on the 17th floor of the Annenberg Pavilion at 100th Street and Madison Avenue. The drab built-to-last stain-resistant hallways leading from the elevator could be part of a research complex anywhere, with windowless laboratories on one side and offices on the other. Signs point the way to biohazard showers. When I entered her office, however, I saw a panorama of Upper Manhattan sloping toward the East River, the water itself, and the Borough of Queens that reminded me of my old office at a bank farther downtown, where the views provided relief from my routine work of writing speeches for senior executives. Until then, it had never quite occurred to me that cutting-edge medical research could be conducted as well as finance in this setting.

Xiu-Min herself welcomed me warmly in her highly accented English, and we made a bit of small talk before I explained my mission, gave her a copy of our book, and asked her to talk about her work, which I had read about in a few newspaper articles.

年后，当我再读这篇文章的时候，当时在学术和实践领域蓬勃发展的中医令我印象深刻。我自己与中医的联系，仅限于在唐人街商店里货架上的罐装干菜。用中医治疗过敏的主意听起来像是用建造金字塔、帕特农神庙和圣保罗大教堂（就更不用说中国自身的任何工程奇迹了）的计划去重建纽约的基础设施。

李秀敏博士的办公室在100号街和麦迪逊大道交叉口处的安纳伯格馆的17楼。从电梯通往任何研究设施的走廊显得单调乏味，经过防污处理。走廊的一侧是没有窗户的实验室，另一侧是办公室。指示牌指向通往生物安全喷淋的方向。然而，当我进到她的办公室的时候，我看到了曼哈顿上城的全景向东河倾斜，这片水和皇后区让我想起了我以前在远离市区的一个银行旁边的老办公室，那个地方的风景可以让我从为高级执行官撰写演讲稿的日常工作中放松下来。我以前从没想过，前沿医学研究可以像在从事金融工作一样的环境下进行。

秀敏用她带着浓重口音的英语热情地欢迎我，我们聊了一会儿，然后我向她说明我的来意。我给了她一本我们的书，并请她给我讲了一下她的工作，我之前在报纸文章上也了解到一些。

She started by explaining that she not only did research but also ran an offsite clinic, treating mostly non-Chinese patients for allergic diseases—many with atopic dermatitis (eczema)—whom traditional allergists couldn't help. Her dream is that Western practitioners will be able to incorporate some of what she does into their work without necessarily learning the secrets of TCM—so-called integrative medicine.

It didn't take long for Dr. Li to convince me that she was on to something. One set of photographs in her computer made an instant impression. From left to right were four views of a little girl's feet. On the left, they were livid with eczema, which, I know from the occasional angry state of my own skin, can itch to the point of obsession. Kids and some grown-ups will scratch until their skin bleeds and gets infected. Paul has told me that when he was a resident at Bellevue, it was not uncommon for children to be hospitalized and their hands tied down to keep their fingers away from their sore skin.

Dr. Li's photographs showed steady improvement. By the third picture, the feet were largely clear, and in the fourth, not only was the skin immaculate, but the nails were polished. As the father of a daughter, I know about the role nail polish can play in a girl's life. The transformation from hated, painful objects to decorative ones was the best indication I could get that something significant had happened.

她首先解释说，她不但做研究，而且在外地开了一个治疗过敏性疾病的诊所，大部分病人都不是中国人，很多病人患有特异性皮炎（湿疹），而传统的过敏症专科医师对于这种病症无能为力。她的梦想是希望西医从业者能够把她所做的一些事情融入自己的工作当中，而无须专门地去学习中医的奥秘——这就是所谓的整合医学。

没多久，李秀敏博士就让我相信了她确实在做些事情。她电脑里的一组照片瞬间给我留下了深刻的印象。从左到右是一个小女孩的脚的四张不同图片。左边的图片上，小女孩的脚是青紫色的，上面有痒得让人抓狂的湿疹，我以前偶尔皮肤出问题时经历过。小孩子和一些成年人会抓自己的皮肤，直到皮肤流血，被感染。保罗曾告诉我，当他还是贝尔维尤医院的住院医生时，经常会看到住院的孩子们被绑住双手，以免手指接触到溃烂的皮肤。

李秀敏博士的照片显示女孩症状的逐步改善。到第三张图片的时候，小女孩的脚大体上已经很干净了。第四张图片中，不但皮肤干净无瑕，而且脚趾涂了指甲油。作为一个女儿的父亲，我知道指甲油在女孩子生活中的重要性。从令人讨厌和痛苦的事物到装饰性的事物，这种转变是我能看到的最好的迹象，表明发生了一些重大的事情。

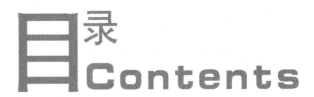

Contents

PART ONE

Background

The first two chapters define the nature of the problem and the context for Dr. Li's research. For many of us, food allergies seem to have come from nowhere, and are often dismissed by those who don't have them as the product of the medical imagination run amok, aided and abetted by indulgent parenting. However, it seems to me that food allergies are not something new, and that the potential for allergies is inherent. It can be elicited by certain interactions between our bodies and the environment, sometimes over generations, and sometimes much faster. The past few decades have seen the steady escalation of provocation to allergies of various kinds, culminating for now with food. Moreover, the medical response has been inadequate to the challenge, emphasizing avoidance, control of symptoms, and the suppression of the immune response. These shortcomings are particularly glaring when the patients are very young children consuming antigens that the rest of us eat with impunity. Times like these cry out for new directions.

❶ An Epidemic of Progress

A child's eczema is usually the initial indication of the medical history that may lie ahead. It is the first step on what allergists call the "atopic [allergic] march" to be followed possibly by environmental allergies, asthma, and food allergies. These conditions seem to be escalating in

第一部分

背　景

本书前两篇定义了食物过敏的性质以及李秀敏博士研究的背景。对于很多人来说，我们似乎并不知道食物过敏的原因是什么，那些没有食物过敏的人经常忽视食物过敏，认为它是医学想象的产物，并受到了父母宠溺教育的煽动和支持。然而，在我看来，食物过敏并不是什么新鲜事，而且潜在的过敏是与生俱来的。过敏可以通过我们身体和环境的相互作用来诱发，有时会跨越几代人（才出现），有时则很快（在一代人身上出现）。各类过敏反应的诱因在过去的几十年间平稳增加，到了现在，食物也会诱发过敏。此外，对于这个挑战，医疗措施尚不充分，强调忌口、控制症状以及抑制免疫反应。当患者是那些非常小的孩子，这些方法的弊端是很明显的，因为那些我们吃了没有问题的食物或药品，对他们来说却是抗原。这样的时代需要新的方向。

❶ 一种发展中的流行病

儿童湿疹通常是未来可能出现的疾病的最初迹象，这是过敏专家所称的"特应性［过敏］进行曲"的第一步，紧随其后的可能就是环境过敏、哮喘和食物过敏。从婴儿潮一代到X

number and severity with each new birth cohort, from baby boomers to generations X and Y, also known as millennials. The apparent explosion of life-threatening food allergies has focused attention on the problem, much of it quite unsympathetic.

Allergies are aggravating to both those who suffer from them and those who resent having to accommodate these patients.

Allergies are an epidemic （lots of people have them） but not a plague, in that they are not communicable and the fatality rates are relatively low. Asthma kills between 3 and 4 thousand Americans every year, and food allergies about 150,[①] many of whom also have asthma.

However, even nonlethal allergies disrupt the lives of children badly enough to make them overtired and inattentive in school, although the children are not usually sick enough to be kept at home. Allergic children are often demoralized to the point that their quality of life is significantly reduced, with long-term effect on learning and participation in normal activities. Similarly, the effect of allergic disease on adults results in reduced productivity and may damage employment prospects. Asthma costs the US economy an estimated ＄56 billion per year in medical outlays and lost productivity at school and work.[②] Allergic rhinitis, which most people call hay fever （although it has nothing to do with either hay or fever）, affects

一代和 Y 一代(也被称为千禧一代)，这些疾病的数量和严重程度似乎都随着每个新出生人群的增加而增加。威胁生命的食物过敏病例的爆发性增长已经吸引了人们的注意,但很多人也显得漠不关心。

对于过敏症患者和那些讨厌但不得不陪伴过敏症患者的人来说,过敏都是非常令人烦恼的。

过敏是流行病(很多人都有),但不是传染病,因为它不具有传染性且致死率相对较低。每年都有 3000 ～ 4000 名美国人死于哮喘,约有 150 人死于过敏,这 150 人中很多人也有哮喘。

然而,过敏就算是不会致命,也严重地破坏了孩子们的生活,因为即使这些孩子通常不会病得严重到要待在家里,他们也会过度疲劳,在学校注意力会不集中。过敏的孩子经常因为他们的生活质量显著降低而沮丧,过敏长期影响他们学习和正常地参与活动。同样地,过敏也影响到成年人,降低他们的生产力并影响他们的就业前景。哮喘每年给美国经济造成约 560 亿美元的医疗负担,并降低学校和产业上的生产力。过敏性鼻炎,很多人称为花粉热(即使它跟花粉和发热都没有关系),影响了

---

① Scott H S. Epidemiology of food allergy[J]. Journal of Allergy and Clinical Immunology, 2001, 127(3):594－602.

② http://www. cdc. gov/media/releases/2011/p0503_vitalsigns. html.

between 10% and 30% of the population worldwide,[①]
costing millions of days of school and work. Among
asthmatic children in the United States, the prevalence
of allergic rhinitis is 61%.[②]

Like other chronic diseases, allergies are stressful
for families. Overseeing the patient's health often
requires drastic alteration in diet and behavior. Siblings
feel slighted, and so do spouses (almost invariably
husbands, because mothers assume the responsibility for
dealing with the allergies). Managing a food-allergic
child costs American families an average of $ 4 000
annually, only 20% of it in medical expenses; the bulk
of the non-medical expenses come in the form of the
sacrifices that parents make at work in order to look
after their children, according to a 2012 survey.[③]

Allergic reactions are prompted not by bacteria or
viruses but by things that present most of us with no ill
effects. Asked to accommodate a seriously allergic
child, the nonallergic are often highly intolerant and
dismissive. As I write this in the days leading up to
Christmas, I have been reading about grandparents,
aunts, and uncles of food-allergic children who would
rather exclude families from holiday feasts than make
considerations in their menus.

The explosive growth of food allergies leads many
people to regard them as something new under the sun.
The refrain from many of my contemporaries is "I
don't remember anyone who was allergic to peanuts
when I was a kid." Come to think of it, I don't

全世界 10% ~ 30% 的人口,占用了
数百万上学日和工作日。在美国患
哮喘的孩子当中,过敏性鼻炎的患病
率是 61%。

过敏像其他的慢性病一样会给
家人带来压力。看护病人让其保持
健康通常需要在饮食和行为上有很
大的改变。兄弟姐妹会感到被忽视,
配偶也是如此(几乎总是丈夫,因为
母亲常承担处理过敏的责任)。根
据 2012 年的一项调查,养育一个食
物过敏孩子的美国家庭平均每年要
花费 4 000 美元,其中只有 20% 是医
疗费用,大部分非医疗费用是父母为
了照顾孩子在工作上做出的牺牲。

过敏反应并不是由细菌或病毒引
起的,而是由对我们大多数人不会产生
不良影响的事物引起的。当被要求容
纳一个严重过敏的孩子时,不过敏的
人往往非常不能容忍和不屑一顾。
当我在圣诞节前夕写这篇文章的时
候,我了解到食物过敏儿童的祖父母、
姑妈和叔伯宁愿不让孩子参加节日
盛宴,也不愿意对菜单进行调整。

食物过敏病例的急剧增长让许
多人将它们视为阳光下的新事物。
我的许多同辈人都说:"当我是个孩
子的时候,我不记得有谁对花生过
敏。"回想起来,我也不记得,但正如

---

① http://www.worldallergy.org/publications/wao_white_book.pdf.

② http://www.ncbi.nlm.nih.gov/pmc/articles/PMC2615278/.

③ Guptaetal.http://www.medpagetoday.com/MeetingCoverage/ACAAI/3594G.

either, but as the author Mark Jackson puts it in his invaluable book, *Allergy: The History of a Modern Malady*,[①] in ancient accounts of reactions to wasp and bee stings, the commonest types of "idiosyncratic reaction" were to foods. He cites the *Hippocratic Corpus*, written four hundred years BCE, which describes a "constituent of the body which is hostile to cheese, and is roused and stirred to action under its influence." Four centuries later, Lucretius wrote, "What is food to one, is to others biting poison." These observers ascribed the reactions to something in the people who reacted, not to the quality of the food. Clearly, the allergic mechanism was always there; it didn't just appear suddenly in 1990.

Allergies are "un-American." All the things that are blamed for the epidemic seem to emanate from our way of life. Greenhouse gases accumulating as fossil fuels are burned are making pollen seasons longer. Asthma gets much worse when the air is full of commerce—diesel particulates, car exhaust, and power-plant emissions. Better standards of sanitation protect us from bacterial infection, but when overdone, they may deprive our immune systems of the challenges they need to keep them in balance; otherwise, useful antibodies then prey on normally harmless proteins. Prolific use of antibiotics kills good bacteria as well as bad ones. Add to this the prevalence of sweet things in children's diets, which may further damage the digestive system, rendering it unable to break down complex proteins that then circulate in the blood as allergens. This indictment of modern living is known

作家马克·杰克逊在他的大作《过敏：一个现代痼疾的历史》中对黄蜂和蜜蜂蜇伤的反应的描述，"特异反应过敏"最常见的类型是食物过敏。他引用了公元前400年的《希波克拉底全集》，书中描述了"对奶酪有敌意的身体成分，被奶酪唤醒和激发去发挥作用"。四个世纪后，卢克莱修写道："吾之美食，汝之鸩毒。"这些观察者把这些反应归因于人体内的某些东西而非归因于食物的质量。显然，过敏机制一直都是存在的，它不是突然在1990年出现的。

过敏是"非美国人特有的"。所有流行病的病因似乎都源于我们的生活方式。随着化石燃料的燃烧，不断积累的温室气体使花粉季节更长。当空气中充满了商业气息，即柴油微粒、汽车尾气和发电厂废气时，哮喘会变得更严重。更好的环境卫生标准可以保护我们免受细菌感染，但当过了头，它们可能会剥夺我们的免疫系统保持平衡所需的挑战；否则，有用的抗体就会捕食那些通常无害的蛋白质。大量使用抗生素在杀死有害的细菌的同时，也会杀死有益的细菌。此外，儿童饮食中普遍存在甜食，这可能会进一步破坏消化系统，使其无法分解复杂的蛋白质，而这些蛋白质随后会成为过敏原在血液中循环。这种对现代生活的"控诉"被

---

① Mark J. Allergy: the history of a modern malady[M]. London: Reaktion Books Ltd., 2006.

broadly as the "hygiene hypothesis."

Food allergens are overwhelmingly found in staples of American diets, especially kids' diets. The big eight allergens are peanuts, tree nuts, milk, eggs, fish, wheat, soy, and shellfish, some of which are frequently hidden in other foods. Peanuts are a special indignity. The anthem of baseball, our national pastime, cries, "Buy me some peanuts and Cracker Jack." Because Cracker Jack has peanuts in it, both of these are a problem to about 1.5% of our children. Jimmy Carter, the only American president since the 19th century to derive any income from agriculture, was in the peanut business. Peanuts are a great source of cheap protein, and that same protein turns out to be hazardous to many children.

New research[①] seems to support the idea that something about the United States makes children more atopic. Immigrant children are less allergic than American children, and having foreign-born parents seems also to afford some protection. The longer these children live in the United States, however, the more allergic they seem to become.

Allergies are not solely an American problem, however. Where "progress" goes, allergies follow, which is something Dr. Susan Prescott observed in her book *The Allergy Epidemic*.[②] Dr. Prescott is from Australia, where the rate of asthma is even higher than it is in the United States and where the financial costs of allergies are double those of arthritis. She contends

广泛称为"健康假设"。

在美国人的日常饮食中,尤其是儿童的饮食中,绝大多数都含有食物过敏原。最主要的八大过敏原是花生、坚果、牛奶、鸡蛋、鱼、小麦、大豆和贝类,其中一些经常隐藏在其他食物中。花生是一种特殊的"伤人尊严"的存在。正如我们的国球——棒球的颂歌里面唱的"给我买一些花生和玉米花生糖"。因为玉米花生糖里有花生,所以花生和玉米花生糖对我们国家1.5%的孩子来说都是问题。吉米·卡特是自19世纪以来唯一一位从农业获得收入的美国总统,他做的就是花生生意。花生是一种廉价蛋白质的重要来源,而事实证明这种蛋白质对许多儿童有危险。

新研究似乎支持了这种观点,即美国的某些方面使儿童更容易出现特应性反应。与美国儿童相比,移民儿童的过敏反应要轻一些,而且父母是在外国出生的儿童对过敏的免疫要强一些。但是,这些孩子在美国生活的时间越长,他们似乎越容易过敏。

然而,过敏不仅仅是美国人的问题。哪里有"发展",过敏就紧跟而来,这是苏珊·普莱斯考特博士在她的《过敏流行病》一书中写到的。普莱斯考特博士来自澳大利亚,在那里哮喘的患病率甚至比美国还高,并且澳大利亚用在过敏上的财政花费是用在关节炎上的两倍。她认为,免疫

---

① Jonathan I S, et al. Prevalence of allergic disease in foreign-born American children[J]. JAMA Pediatrics, 2013, 167(6): 554-560.

② Susan P. The allergy epidemic[M]. Washington: UWA Publishing, 2011.

that the immune system has adjusted to the modern world by subtle changes in DNA that cause it to treat otherwise harmless proteins as lethal intruders："As allergic reactions are directed to the external environment, it makes sense that the areas of the body affected are those that are in most immediate contact with the environment：the skin, the airways and the gut." Thus, the allergic march—eczema, nasal allergies, asthma, and food allergies；as countries industrialize, these diseases march forward together.

Basics of Allergy

I will explain some of the basics of allergy now because the concepts are crucial for understanding what happens throughout the remainder of the book.

The word "allergy" was coined by the Viennese doctor Clemens von Pirquet in 1906 from the Greek *allos*, which means "different" or "other," and *ergon*, connoting energy or reactivity. [①]

The ability to distinguish things that belong in your body from those that don't is the foundation of the immune system. The immune system is not one thing but really a group of interlocking subsystems whose beneficial functions sometimes turn around and bite us. There are two principal components, the first being the *innate* immune system, which fights invaders but doesn't "remember" them. That is, each time the innate immune system encounters an infectious microbe or virus, it will attack it the same way, even if the body has been exposed repeatedly.

系统为了适应现代社会,在 DNA 上有了微妙的变化,这些变化导致免疫系统把无害的蛋白质作为致命的入侵者去对待:"由于过敏反应是直接针对外部环境的,那么身体上受影响的区域都是与环境有最直接接触的地方:皮肤,呼吸道和肠道。"因此,过敏也在发展——湿疹、鼻过敏、哮喘和食物过敏;随着国家工业化的发展,这些疾病也在一同发展。

过敏的基本知识

我现在将解释过敏的一些基本知识,因为这些概念对于理解这本书的其余部分至关重要。

Allergy(过敏)一词是维也纳医生克莱门斯·冯·皮尔凯在 1906 年创造的,来自希腊语中的"allos"和"ergon",前者表示"不同的"或"其他",后者意味着能量或反应。

区分属于你身体的东西和不属于你身体的东西的能力是免疫系统的基础。免疫系统不是一个东西,而是一组相互关联的子系统,其有益的功能有时会反过来伤害到我们。免疫系统主要有两个组成部分,第一个是先天性免疫系统,它会对抗"侵略者",但不会"记住"他们。也就是说,每当先天性免疫系统遇到一个感染性的细菌或者病毒,它就会用同样的方式攻击它,即使身体已经反复地暴露于那些细菌和病毒。

---

① Jackson, op cit., p. 27.

The other part is the *adaptive* immune system. This is the part that we learned about in high school. A first exposure to a virus such as smallpox can be deadly, but if by some miracle we survive, such a virus won't present a problem because we will have created antibodies that will recognize the virus and mobilize defenses that will kill it before it kills us. Dr. Jerome Groopman describes "the elegant choreography of [the T cells]…coordinating scores of enzymes and releasing a repertoire of proteins that, in the body, amounts to a solid wall of immune defense."①

Allergic reactions are a function of the adaptive system.

At the time of a *primary exposure* to an allergen, the immune system reacts in one of three ways, two of which are positive or harmless and the third of which is allergic. There are two kinds of helper T cells that come into play. These are Th1 cells (T-helper 1), which are associated with tolerance to allergens, and Th2 cells (T-helper 2), which are associated with allergies. They signal to B cells, another class of white blood cells or lymphocytes, to produce antibodies called *immunoglobulins*, via a set of proteins called *cytokines*. The B cells are individually programmed to recognize a single antibody for a single antigen. When they get signals from Th1 cells, they produce an antibody called immunoglobulin G, or IgG. On our website we call it IgG[ood]. Th2 cells regulate production of the antibody IgE, or IgE[vil]. Both IgE and IgG are allergen specific. That is, each antibody is

另一个部分是适应性免疫系统。这部分我们在高中时已经学过。首次接触像天花这样的病毒可能是致命的,但如果我们奇迹般地生存了下来,像这样的病毒对我们来说就不再是问题了,因为我们的身体已经创造出了能识别那种病毒的抗体,并且那些抗体会调动防御系统在病毒杀死我们之前杀死病毒。杰罗姆·古罗柏曼博士描述道,"(T 细胞)优雅地组合起来,协调大量酶,释放出一系列蛋白质,在体内相当于一道坚实的免疫防御墙。"

过敏反应是适应性免疫系统的一种功能。

在初次接触过敏原的时候,免疫系统会作出三种反应,其中两种是积极无害的,第三种就是过敏。有两类辅助性 T 细胞会起作用。它们是与过敏原的耐受性有关的辅助性 T 细胞 1(Th1 细胞)和与过敏有关的辅助性 T 细胞 2(Th2 细胞)。它们通过一组称为细胞因子的蛋白质给 B 细胞发信号,B 细胞是另一类白细胞或淋巴细胞,可以产生被称为免疫球蛋白的抗体。B 细胞分别被编程,以识别针对单一抗原的单一抗体。当它们从 Th1 细胞那里得到信号,它们会产生一种叫作免疫球蛋白 G(IgG)的抗体。在我们的网站上,我们称它为[好]IgG。Th2 细胞调节抗体 IgE 或者[坏]IgE 的产生。IgE 和 IgG 具有过敏原特异性。也就是说,每一个抗体都被编程为对单一过

---

① Jerome G. How doctors think[M]. UK: Mariner Books, 2008: 122.

programmed to respond to a single allergen.

These antibodies bind themselves to receptors on *effector* cells—mainly *mast cells* (discovered in 1878 by, as we call him in our family, "the other Dr. Paul Ehrlich"—no relation) and *basophils*. The mast cells lodge primarily in the tissues where they are likely to encounter outside agents the skin, sinuses, lungs, and digestive tract. The *basophils* circulate in the blood.

Think of all the classic signs of an immune response in, say, a pimple that sprouts overnight—the redness and swelling caused by the release of fluid from the blood vessels in the region, pain as increased swelling stimulates local pain fibers, and heat. The body is trying to isolate and combat an infection from a clogged pore.

Then picture this same process happening inside you. When IgE-equipped cells encounter their target allergen, the chain of events we associate with an allergy attack commences. The mast cells release a "soup" of substances called *mediators* to attack it, the best known of which is histamine. When all this happens in your sinuses, you sneeze and get congested. When it happens in your lungs, you wheeze. With food allergies left untreated for even a few minutes, the process unfolds unpredictably in different parts of the body. An innocuous protein precipitates a full-scale inflammatory response. It's like calling 9-1-1 when your teenager forgets his house key and tries to enter the house through a basement window in the middle of the night: Once the cops arrive, mistakes can be made.

敏原作出反应。

这些抗体在效应细胞上与受体相结合,这些效应细胞主要是肥大细胞(在1878年被"另一个保罗·埃尔利希博士"发现的,在我们的家庭中是这样叫他的,和我们无血缘关系)和嗜碱性粒细胞。肥大细胞主要存在于皮肤、鼻窦、肺和消化道等可能遇到外源性因素的组织中。嗜碱性粒细胞在血液中循环。

想一下免疫反应的所有典型特征,例如,一夜之间长出的痘痘——由该区域血管中释放的液体所引起的红肿,由于逐步增加的肿胀刺激局部疼痛纤维所造成的痛和热。这是身体正试图通过一个堵塞的毛孔去隔离感染并与之做斗争。

然后想象一下同样的过程发生在你的身体内。当配备IgE的细胞遇到目标过敏原,与过敏发作相关的一系列事件就开始了。肥大细胞释放一种称为"介质"的液体物质来攻击它,其中最广为人知的是组胺。当所有的这些都发生在你的鼻窦里时,你会打喷嚏、鼻塞。当它发生在你的肺里时,你会喘息。如果食物过敏不及时治疗即便只是几分钟,身体的不同部位就会展开不可预知的反应。一种无害的蛋白质骤然引发一场全面的炎症反应。这就像是在半夜的时候,你十几岁的孩子忘记带房子的钥匙了,然后他试图通过地下室的窗户进入房子,结果有人打了911报警电话:一旦警察到达,就会出现误会。

Three Responses to Primary Exposure Occur

First is *immunization*. That is, the immune system will recognize an allergen but will react by producing IgG, courtesy of Th1, overwhelmingly a benign, protective antibody response against viruses such as smallpox and polio or bacteria, specifically a so-called blocking antibody called IgG4, which attaches itself to your effector cells. If your effector cells are equipped with allergen-specific IgG4, they will not release their toxins in the event that they encounter this allergen. There are tests available that show the presence of allergen-specific IgG. These do not mean you have an allergy (although there are those who contend otherwise, mostly vendors of fringe tests and therapies); they merely signify that you have been exposed.

Second is *tolerance*. There will be no clinical symptoms because the body can simply coexist with the substance, a kind of physiological "don't ask, don't tell" policy. Sometimes there is an initial immune response that becomes less and less with repeated exposures.

Third is *sensitization*. This response results from overproduction of the antibody IgE and a lack of regulation of the inflammatory response. It should be noted that high serum IgE levels—i. e., antibodies circulating in the blood—are not indicative of an allergy. They become a problem only if, as described above, they are mounted on effector cells. Normally, IgE should be the least abundant antibody in the blood—0. 05% of all immunoglobulins.[①] A highly

---

① http://en. wikipedia. 0rg/wiki/Immunoglobulin_E#cite_ref-8.

初次接触的三种反应

第一种是免疫。即免疫系统会识别一个过敏原并由Th1产生IgG作出反应,绝大多数是针对天花和脊髓灰质炎病毒或细菌的良性、保护性抗体反应,特别是所谓的阻断抗体IgG4,它会附着到你的效应细胞上。如果你的效应细胞配备有过敏原特异性IgG4,在它们遇到这种过敏原时就不会释放毒素。有些测试可以表明存在过敏原特异性IgG。但并非说明你已经患有过敏症(尽管有些人持反对意见,大多数是提供边缘检验和疗法的供应商),而仅仅表明你已经接触了过敏原。

第二种是耐受。在这种反应中没有临床症状,因为身体可以与这些物质和平共处,一种生理上的"不问,不说"原则。有时,初始的免疫反应会随着重复接触而变得越来越少。

第三种是致敏。这种反应源于IgE抗体生产过剩和炎症反应缺乏调节。应注意高水平的免疫血清IgE——比如,抗体在血液中循环并不代表过敏。只有当如上所述,它们附着在效应细胞上时,才会成为问题。通常,IgE应该是血液中最少的抗体,占所有免疫球蛋白的0.05%。严重过敏的人,体内IgE的含量是不

allergic individual will have many times more IgE than a nonallergic person. All those idle hands and so few natural enemies! The IgE antibodies don't have enough to do and start to recognize otherwise harmless or beneficial proteins as the enemy. The allergenic proteins associated with most serious reactions—Ara h1, 2, and 3① are the hardest to digest. They can withstand the onslaught of acids and enzymes that break down other proteins, including the weaker allergens Ara h6 and 8, gain access to the rest of the body through the stomach and the intestines, and possibly spark devastating reactions. ②

It turns out that Ara h1 protein in peanuts is found in other things, including parasitic worms and insect venom, which provoke the immune system. Why do certain proteins end up in such disparate organisms? These shared elements are called "common protein domains," which are "part of a given protein sequence and structure that can evolve, function, and exist independently of the rest of the protein chain. "③ These common protein domains can also be plucked from one organism and grafted into the DNA of another, the basis of genetic modification, which frightens many of us, especially those with food-allergic children. Common protein domains have been identified in a variety of parasites, in multiple animal species, including cats, dogs, and people, and in plant

过敏的人的很多倍。闲置的抗体太多,而天敌太少了! IgE 抗体没事做,就开始把其他无害或有益的蛋白质当作敌人了。与最严重的反应相关联的致敏蛋白——Ara h1,2 和 3 是最难消化的。它们可以承受那些能够分解其他蛋白质的酸和酶的攻击,包括较弱的过敏原 Ara h6 和 8,通过肠胃进入到身体的其他部位,就有可能引发毁灭性的反应。

原来,花生中含有的 Ara h1 蛋白也存在于其他事物中,包括寄生虫和昆虫毒液,这些都会刺激免疫系统。为何某些蛋白质会存在于不同的生物体中呢? 原因是这些生物体享有同一种"常见蛋白质结构域"。这种蛋白质结构域是已知蛋白序列和结构的一部分,可以独立于剩余蛋白质肽链而进化、作用和存在。这些常见的蛋白质结构域也可以从一个有机体移植到另一个 DNA 上,这是基因改造的基础,令许多人尤其是那些有食物过敏的孩子恐惧。常见的蛋白质结构域已经在多种寄生虫,多个包括猫狗在内的动物物种、人类和植物物种中得到识别。

---

① Short for aracbis bypogaea, Greek for "peanut. "

　全称为 aracbis bypogaea,希腊语,表示"花生"。

② Soheila J M, Si-Yin C, Elaine T C, et al. The effects of roasting on the allergenic properties of peanut proteins[J]. Journal of Allergy and Clinical Immunology, 2000, 106(4): 763－768.

③ http://en. wikipedia. org/wiki/Protein_domain.

species. [1]

Why do these proteins survive evolution? Let's just say they are there for a reason, such as storing energy or protecting from predators. Nature doesn't like to reinvent the wheel, either. Somewhere along the evolutionary continuum, these building blocks of life stayed the same even as some microorganisms diverged into plants and animals.

为什么这些蛋白质能在进化中存活下来？让我们假设它们的存在是有原因的，比如储存能量或者保护自己不受捕食者的伤害。大自然也不喜欢白费力气做重复的工作。在进化的连续性上，即使一些微生物分化成植物和动物，这些生命的组成部分仍然保持不变。

Origins of an Epidemic

一种流行病的起源

Why have allergies increased exponentially in the past few generations? A new science called epigenetics is key to understanding what has happened, referring to "heritable changes in gene expression that are not due to changes in the DNA sequence". Subtle alterations in gene expression—what genes do and when they do them—are likely influenced by changes in environmental exposures. Genes themselves comprise only 2% of the genome, but the rest of the genome—which has been called "junk DNA"—contributes to the development of any organism in ways that have only recently come into focus. [2]

为什么过敏在过去几代急剧增加？一个被称为表观遗传学的新科学是理解发生了什么的关键，它指的是"基因表达的变化，而不是DNA序列的变化。"微妙的基因表达的改变（基因表达什么，什么时候表达）很有可能受环境变化的影响。基因本身只占基因组的2%，但其余被称为"垃圾DNA"的基因组有助于任何生物的发展，这也只是最近才引起人们的关注。

Some researchers describe the *epigenome* as the "clothing" of the genome, in which "certain layers change significantly during development and can be modified throughout life, whereas other layers remain relatively permanent". These differences help explain why individuals with the same or similar DNA—

一些研究人员把表观基因组描述为基因组的"衣服"，其中"某些层在发展过程中会发生显著的变化，并且在整个生命过程当中都可以被改造，而其他层保持相对的永久性"。这些差异有助于解释为什么具有相

---

① Bielory B P, John T, Bielory L. Allergic reactions to common allergens may be due to evolutionary immune response to conserved domains (CDs) present in parasites and allergens[J]. Journal of Allergy and Clinical Immunology, 2006, 117 (2): SI17.

② Kiyoshi H, Amanda P, Gol- naz V, et al. Mechanisms underlying helper T-cell plasticity: implications for immune-mediated disease[J]. Journal of Allergy and Clinical Immunology, 2013, 131(5): 1276-1287.

identical or unidentical twins, for example—may have very different health outcomes. Two important mechanisms contribute to this process by essentially sticking chemical "tags" on the DNA or the proteins that surround it, called *histones*. Methyl groups can be added to the DNA (this is called DNA methylation), which generally switches the gene "off," or histones can be chemically modified by the addition of acetyl groups, which leads to greater expression of the DNA. Conversely, the removal of methyl groups from DNA (demethylation) and acetyl groups from histones (deacetylation) switches genes "on." [1]

Families may be programmed by their DNA not to be allergy prone, but changes in gene expression can undermine that protection. Versions of this happen at each intersection of the body and the environment, as Dr. Prescott pointed out, and the changes in one generation can be passed to succeeding generations. UCLA researchers John S. Torday and Virender K. Rehan have found what they call a "smoking gun" linking grandmothers' smoking to asthma in their grandchildren. [2]

People who itch and sneeze seem to have children who wheeze, who then seem to have children who hive, swell up, collapse from plunging blood pressure, and asphyxiate upon eating certain foods.

Allergy treatment has generally been directed at symptoms, not at root causes. We take antihistamines

同或相似 DNA 的个体——比如同卵或异卵双胞胎——或许会有非常不同的健康状况。本质上是通过在 DNA 或其周围的蛋白质上贴上化学"标签",两个重要的机制有助于这一过程的完成,它们本质上是将化学"标签"贴在 DNA 或其周围的蛋白质(称为组蛋白)上。甲基团可以添加到 DNA 上(这被称为 DNA 甲基化),一般会"关掉"基因,或组蛋白可以通过添加乙酰基基团从而被化学改良,这可以引起 DNA 更强的表达。相反,把甲基团从 DNA 上移除(去甲基化)或者把乙酰基基团从组蛋白上移除(去乙酰化),会"开启"基因。

家庭成员可以通过 DNA 编辑变得不容易过敏,但基因表达的变化会破坏这种保护。这种情况发生在身体和环境的每一个交叉点上,正如普雷斯科特博士指出的那样,一代人的变化可以传给下几代人。加州大学洛杉矶分校(UCLA)的研究人员约翰·S.托迪和维兰德·K.雷汗发现了其所称的祖母吸烟和孙辈患哮喘之间联系的"确凿证据"。

有瘙痒和打喷嚏毛病的人的孩子似乎会气喘、起荨麻疹、肿胀,会因为血压的急剧下降而体力不支,并且会因为吃了某些食物而窒息。

过敏治疗通常是治标不治本。我们打喷嚏的时候会用抗组胺,气喘

① http://www. asthma- allergieschildren. com/2012/11/06/do-allergies-develop-in-the-womb/.

② John S T, Virender K R. An epigenetic "smoking gun" for reproductive inheritance[J]. Expert Review of Obstetrics & Gynecology, 2013, 8(2): 99-101.

when we sneeze and inhaled albuterol when we wheeze and try to steer clear of our triggers—the specific allergens that make us sick. Sometimes we use medicines prophylactically, such as antihistamines starting before the pollen season and inhaled corticosteroids to keep asthmatic inflammation under control, reducing the chance of an attack. (The inability to cure most allergies has made the pharmaceutical industry the center of a battle that long predates current frustration at the lack of progress; for a detailed account, see Mark Jackson's book.)

The closest we have to a cure is *hyposensitization*, consisting of multiyear programs *of immunotherapy*—also called allergy shots—which have been used to treat allergies for more than a century. The shots begin with small doses of antigen/allergen—a fraction of a unit—which are gradually increased until they reach a maximum or a maintenance dose. As IgE production is continually activated by introduction of the antigen, the cells that regulate production of new IgE (Th2 cells) are widely thought to become overloaded, and the quantity of IgE circulating diminishes proportionately with the amount of IgG4, the blocking antibody. As immunotherapy continues, these benign antibodies compete with IgE for available receptor sites on new mast cells in a kind of game of musical chairs, although once the antibodies are "seated," they don't get up again. Over time, with turnover of effector cells, the benign IgG antibodies dominate and allergenicity subsides. Now, another mode of therapy called *sublingual immunotherapy*—frequently called SLIT—in which the allergens are placed under the tongue, is growing in popularity, the idea of which

的时候吸入沙丁胺醇治疗,并且试图避开我们的触发物,即那些会使我们生病的特定的过敏原。有时我们使用药物进行预防,如在花粉季节开始前使用抗组胺药,及吸入皮质类固醇激素使哮喘炎症得到控制,减少发作的机会。(制药业由于不能治愈大多数过敏而成为争论的焦点,这场争论未取得任何进展,早就陷入了当下的沮丧;更详细的解释,请看马克·杰克逊的书。)

我们最接近治愈的疗法是由多年的免疫治疗计划组成的脱敏——也称为过敏疫苗注射——它被用于治疗过敏已有一个多世纪。注射从开始用小剂量的抗原/过敏原到一个单元的一小部分再逐渐增加,直到最大并维持剂量。由于免疫球蛋白IgE的产生是通过抗原的引入而不断被激活的,所以人们普遍认为调节新IgE(Th2细胞)产生的细胞已经超负荷,并随着阻断性抗体IgG4量的积累,循环的免疫球蛋白IgE的数量也随之减少。随着免疫疗法的继续,这些良性抗体就像在玩抢板凳的游戏,为了附着在新肥大细胞的可用受体上而与免疫球蛋白进行竞争,抗体一旦"坐下"后,它们绝不再起来。随着时间的推移和效应细胞的转换,良性的免疫球蛋白抗体开始占据主导,过敏逐渐消退。现在,另一种名为舌下免疫治疗的疗法——通常被称为免疫治疗——过敏原被放置在舌下正越来越受欢迎,因为父母发现

parents find attractive for their kids. However, European doctors are more accepting of it than Americans. There are, moreover, reasons to doubt its effectiveness. ①②

Shots haven't succeeded with food allergies, however. People with the worst food allergies are so sensitive that administration of even minute quantities of the allergen can provoke a deadly systemic response. That is what makes food allergies such a daily horror for millions of families. The big-eight food allergens are not only practically ubiquitous in standard American diets in their recognizable forms but are commodity additives to thousands of processed foods. A nonallergic child who eats tuna fish every day for lunch may be vulnerable from long-term exposure to mercury, but a dairy-allergic child also has to watch out for the milk protein casein that is sometimes added as a preservative.

Currently, numerous trials are underway at several research centers, usually coordinated under the Consortium of Food Allergy Research [COFAR]③ because of the difficulty of finding enough patients to take part, for courses of oral immunotherapy (OIT) for food allergies, an idea with a hundred-year history, in which escalating doses are consumed. (The Jaffe Food Allergy Institute at Mount Sinai in New York, where Dr. Li works, is prominent in these trials.) It remains to be seen, however, if the OIT trials, which

这种疗法对孩子很有吸引力。然而，欧洲的医生比美国医生更能接受这种疗法。当然，有理由怀疑其有效性。

然而，疫苗注射在食物过敏上没有成功过。患有严重食物过敏的人们非常敏感，即使摄入微量的过敏原都可能引发致命的全身反应。这就是为什么食物过敏使数百万家庭每天都经历着恐惧。八大类食品过敏原不仅几乎无处不以可识别的形式存在于标准美国饮食中，还存在于成千上万的加工食品添加剂中。每天午餐都吃金枪鱼的非过敏儿童可能由于长期摄入汞而变得脆弱，且乳品过敏的孩子也要注意有时作为防腐剂添加的牛奶蛋白酪蛋白。

目前，几个研究中心正在进行的众多试验通常是在食物过敏研究联盟（COFAR）的协调下进行，因为很难找到足够的患者参加食物过敏的口服免疫疗法（OIT）。OIT 具有百年历史，其间消耗了大量药物。（李秀敏博士工作的纽约西奈山的贾菲食品过敏研究所在这些试验中表现突出。）然而，OIT 试验虽然对一些患

① Danilo D B, Antonella P, Maria S L B, et al. Efficacy of subcutaneous and sublingual immunotherapy with grass allergens for seasonal allergic rhinitis: a meta-analysis-based comparison[J]. Journal of Allergy and Clinical Immunology, 2012, 130(5): 1097-1107.

② Menno A K, Esther R, Roy G van W, et al. Real-Life compliance and persistence among users of subcutaneous and sublingual allergen immunotherapy[J]. Journal of Allergy and Clinical Immunology, 2013, 132(2): 353-360.

③ https://web.emmes.com/study/cofar/.

have been promising for some patients, will result in lasting clinical unresponsiveness, as is the case with environmental allergy shots, or will have to be supplemented perpetually by regular doses of the allergen (as with insect venom immunotherapy). Mothers I correspond with say that their children will have to take eight peanuts a day for the rest of their lives after "completing" their OIT. The stakes are high. When seasonal allergens return, they are annoying; when anaphylaxis returns, the consequences can be tragic.

As Dr. Li puts it, "OIT doesn't fundamentally alter the immune system. The Th2 cells that regulate production of IgE may be stimulated to produce it until they are worn out, but new ones are created all the time. Without new allergen exposure to exhaust their IgE output in early stages, they may regain their strength." This happens with other forms of immunotherapy, such as rush immunotherapy for penicillin. When penicillin-allergic patients need antibiotics, they can be desensitized rapidly, which works long enough to receive treatment, but afterward, they will still be allergic and would require the same regimen the next time they need penicillin. It's one thing to receive rush immunotherapy, which you only need temporarily for an isolated medical procedure,[①] and another to spend months and months doing OIT for foods.

The distinction between desensitization and cure is critical. OIT may effectively raise the threshold of

者来说有效,但是否会带来持久的临床无反应,或者像环境过敏注射一样必须永久补充常规剂量的过敏原(如昆虫毒液免疫疗法),还有待观察。和我保持联系的妈妈们说她们的孩子在"完成"OIT 后,以后每天必须吃八颗花生。这个风险很高,季节性过敏原返回时是令人烦恼的;当过敏性反应复发时,后果可能是悲剧性的。

正如李秀敏博士所说,"OIT 不能从根本上改变免疫系统。调节 IgE 产生的 Th2 细胞可能会被刺激产生 IgE,直到它们耗尽为止,但是新的 Th2 细胞一直在产生。如果 Th2 细胞在早期阶段没有被出现的新过敏原耗尽 IgE 的产生,他们可能重新产生过敏。"这种情况也发生在其他形式的免疫疗法上,如青霉素快速免疫疗法。当青霉素过敏的患者需要抗生素时,青霉素可以让他们迅速脱敏,脱敏时间足够长来接受治疗,但之后,他们仍然会对青霉素过敏,下一次需要青霉素时也需要同样的治疗方案。接受快速免疫疗法就是这样,你只需要暂时进行一个隔离的医疗程序,而 OIT 要花数月的时间来寻找合适的食物。

区别脱敏和治愈是至关重要的。OIT 可以有效地提高反应的阈值来

---

① Paul M E. Asthma allergies children: a parent's guide[M]. New York: Third Avenue Books, 2010.

reactivity to reduce the possibility of accidental exposure, but whether it will permanently end the need for vigilance that food-allergic kids and their parents practice every day remains to be seen. Until it is, they must read labels minutely, avoid most restaurants, and carry powerful medication everywhere they go, all the behaviors that make food allergies so burdensome.

Another problem is that because IgE is allergen specific, it's hard to treat a patient for more than one food allergy at a time because of the danger of a serious reaction—one allergen may be tolerated fine and the other a problem, and the doctor wouldn't know which was which. That's why most of the studies of OIT are for only one allergen at a time (except for those studies that also use an "anti-IgE" medicine call Xolair—aka omalizumab—which costs $1 000 a month and up for use with asthma). If, instead of desensitizing to one allergen at a time, we can modulate IgE in general until it is reduced to a normal, healthy fraction of immunoglobulin output, we would be much closer to a cure for food allergies while simultaneously treating "IgE-mediated" eczema, asthma, and environmental allergies.

An additional factor may be that anti-IgE omalizumab reduces the density of the high-affinity receptors on mast cells and basophils and makes them less sensitive to allergens. [1]

Dr. Li's research concentrates on the modulation side of that divide. She says, "We want to turn bad

减少意外接触的可能,但它是否会永久性地结束食物过敏儿童及其父母每天对过敏的警惕,仍有待观察。在得到确认之前,他们必须详细阅读食物标签,规避大多数餐馆并且随身携带强有效的药物,所有这些行为都让食物过敏变得不堪忍受。

另一个问题是,由于 IgE 具有过敏原特异性,所以一次治疗只能针对病人对一种食物的过敏症状,因为其严重反应的危险性——一种过敏原可以耐受良好,另一种却是问题,医生也分不清楚是哪种食物过敏。这就是为什么大多数 OIT 的研究每次只针对一种过敏原(除了那些也使用叫作奥马珠单抗——阿卡·奥马珠单抗的"抗 IgE"药物的研究,该药用于哮喘,每月花费 1000 美元以上)。如果不是一次只对一种过敏原脱敏,我们一般可以调节 IgE,直到它被降低到免疫球蛋白输出的正常的健康部分,我们将更可能治愈食物过敏,同时治疗 IgE 介导的湿疹、哮喘和环境过敏。

一个额外的因素可能是抗 IgE 的奥马珠单抗降低在肥大细胞和嗜碱性粒细胞上高亲和性受体的密度,降低它们对过敏原的敏感度。

李秀敏博士的研究集中在分化的调节方面。她说,"我们想把坏男

① Tse Wen C, Yu-Yu S. Anti-IgE as a mast cell-stabilizing therapeutic agent [J]. Journal of Allergy and Clinical Immunology, 2006, 117(6): 1203 - 1212.

boys into good boys. " She told me at that initial meeting two years ago, "It's not too early to talk about a cure. " That was a surprise to me, because from everything I had read, it was far too early. Moreover, the fact that she was basing her research on combinations of herbs hundreds or even thousands of years old was counter to my own intuitions and ethnocentric biases. My conception of this kind of medicine was shaped by this exchange between Carl Reiner and Mel Brooks playing his classic character the 2000-Year-Old Man:

Reiner: What did you do to stay healthy?

Brooks: We had herbs, certain grasses, certain barks of certain trees…which are not to be mentioned on this record.

Reiner: Why not?

Brooks: Because I don't want to throw the entire ethical drug industry into chaos! Little did I know.

Dr. Li spent five years starting in the late 1970s, not long after the universities were reopened, getting an MD in a Chinese medical school in Zhengzhou, where she studied both Chinese and Western medicines, and then another three years studying integrative clinical pediatric immunology in Beijing. After a year at Stanford, she had three years of additional training in clinical immunology at Johns Hopkins Medical School, working with Dr. Hugh Sampson. Dr. Sampson has been a leading figure in the effort to comprehend and treat the food-allergy epidemic since the 1980s. At Johns Hopkins, he led the effort to isolate the allergenic proteins in peanuts from 30 down to seven, among other things, and research into the possibility of injectable immunotherapy. Dr. Sampson

孩变成好男孩。"她在两年前的首次会议上告诉我,"现在谈论治愈方法已经不算太早。"这对我来说是一个惊喜,因为从我读过的一切来看,这太超前了。此外,她把研究建立在几百年甚至几千年前的草药组合上的事实与我自己的直觉和种族中心偏见背道而驰。我对这种药物的概念是从卡尔·赖纳和梅尔·布鲁克斯在有关后者所扮演的 2 000 岁老人这一经典角色进行交流中所得来的:

赖纳:你做了什么来保持健康?

布鲁克斯:我们有草药,某些草,某些树的某种树皮……这些在这个采访上不能被提到。

赖纳:为什么不呢?

布鲁克斯:因为我不想把整个处方药品行业搞乱,我知道的太少。

李秀敏博士从 20 世纪 70 年代末期开始,即中国恢复高考不久之后,花费了五年时间,在位于郑州的一所中医学院学习中西医并获得医学学士学位,然后又在北京学习了三年的综合临床儿科免疫学。在斯坦福大学学习一年后,她与休·桑普森博士合作,在约翰·霍普金斯医学院接受了三年的临床免疫学培训。桑普森博士是自 20 世纪 80 年代以来致力于理解和治疗食物过敏流行病的领军人物。在约翰·霍普金斯大学,他领导了一项工作,将花生过敏性原蛋白质从 30 种降到了 7 种,并

is currently chief of the Division of Allergy & Immunology in the Department of Pediatrics, director of the Jaffe Food Allergy Institute, and dean of Translational Biomedical Science at the Mount Sinai Medical Center. He is also past president of the American Academy of Allergy, Asthma, and Immunology（AAAAI）. His eventual decision to support Dr. Li's ideas may prove to be a pivotal event in the direction of allergy research and treatment.

After I met Dr. Li, I tried to get into the spirit of things and spent a few months reading about TCM with its thousands of years of tradition, belief systems, and alternative anatomy. I was bored. I don't believe that people can channel Qi（pronounced *chee*）and knock me over from across the room. And a philosophy that seems to boil down to "everything in moderation"— well, life is too short. Mine is, anyway.

The medical part of TCM is something else, though. In TCM literature, the formulas are directed at specific body parts and exhaustively described symptoms. They are also evocatively and poetically named; for example, the essential text *Formulas and Strategies* lists Cool the Bones Powder, which "clears heat from deficiency and alleviates steaming bone disorder," as does Sweet Wormwood and Soft-Shelled Turtle Shell Decoction Version 1.[①]（I wonder what the people responsible for names like Avastin and Celebrex would do with these medicines.）

研究了注射免疫治疗的可能性。桑普森博士目前是儿科部过敏与免疫部主任,贾菲食品过敏研究所主任,西奈山医学中心转化生物医学科学中心主任,也是美国过敏、哮喘和免疫学会（AAAAI）的前主席。他最终决定支持李秀敏博士的想法,这可能是过敏研究和治疗方向上的一个关键事件。

在见到李秀敏博士之后,我试图深入了解中医药的内涵,花了几个月的时间阅读有关中医的数千年的传统、理念体系和替代解剖学。我感到它很无趣。因为我不相信人类可以发出强大的气流并将房间另一头的我打翻在地,以及一种似乎可以归结为"一切都要适度"的哲学——好吧,生命太短暂了。不管怎么说,我的也是。

但是中医的药物部分不一样。在中医文献中,方剂只针对特定身体部位及详尽描述的症状。其命名也令人回味并具有诗意。比如,在《方剂和疗法》中讲到清骨散,甜蒿和软壳龟壳汤剂组方1,它"清虚热,减轻骨蒸症状"。（我在想那些为如安维汀和西乐葆这些药起名的人们会用这些药做什么。）

---

① Volker S, Dan B, Andrew E, et al. Chinese Herbal Medicine Formulas & Strategies[M]. 2nd ed. Seattle：Eastland Press, 2009.

If we can connect the classical TCM formulas with pathology recognized by Western doctors, we may get a head start on finding cures. As Dr. Scott Sicherer, professor of pediatrics and chief of Pediatric Allergy and Immunology at Mount Sinai School of Medicine, told me, "In China, what we call traditional Chinese medicine is just medicine. Western medicine looks at individual molecules to treat specific conditions, but it may be that many molecules or ingredients can do better and can affect the larger immune system. By looking at them one at a time, we may be missing out."

Enter Dr. Li.

The Ancient Origins of a "Modern" Affliction

We associate allergies with the industrialized world, but although the incidence of allergic diseases has increased exponentially over the past few generations, these tendencies have been there all along. When the Yellow Emperor began collecting remedies from Chinese doctors three thousand years ago, they were already treating symptoms that sound like allergies, and these remedies are still in use today. You don't have to believe that Prometheus brought fire from the heavens to know that you can use it to boil water.

Dr. Li sits between the two traditions like a Rosetta Stone, providing the key to translating the ancient into the modern. Studying her work and speaking to her colleagues, it's hard for me to escape the impression that she is a pivotal figure in medicine. She embodies a saying given to me by a Chinese-speaking friend: *tianshi*, *dili*, *renhe* (heavenly timing,

如果我们可以将中医经方与西医医生认可的病理学联系起来,我们可能会在找到治愈方法上得到优势。西奈山医学院儿科学教授兼儿科过敏与免疫学主任斯科特·史可瑞博士告诉我:"在中国,我们所说的中医就是医学。西医着眼于单独的分子来治疗特定的病症,但(着眼于)许多分子或成分可能会做得更好,可以影响更大的免疫系统。如果我们每次只着眼于一个分子或成分,我们可能会错失良机。"

走近李秀敏博士。

"现代"痛苦的古代起源

我们将过敏与工业化世界联系起来,尽管过敏性疾病的发病率在过去几代人中急剧增长,其实这种趋势一直存在。当黄帝在三千年前开始从中医医生那里收集治疗方法时,他们已经在治疗听起来像过敏的症状,而且这些治疗方法至今仍在使用。你不必相信火是普罗米修斯从天堂带来的,但你可以用火来煮开水。

李秀敏博士就像一块罗塞塔石碑,竖在中西医两种传统之间,为古今转换提供了钥匙。研究她的工作并与她的同事交谈,我很难不产生这样的印象:她是医学界的关键人物。她体现了一个华人朋友对我说的话:天时地利人和。我

location advantage, and human harmony), or, as we put it, being in the right place at the right time. I believe that if it hadn't been for the unique attributes of this individual, the integration of Western medicine and TCM would never have gotten as far as it has in this country, and, because she is so active on various national and international committees devoted to complementary and alternatives medicine, maybe in the world.

Dr. Julie Wang, one of Xiu-Min's colleagues at Mount Sinai who serves with her on those committees, is second-generation Taiwanese American. She was born and raised in the United States and educated in an American medical school. She said her only acquaintance with TCM was when she was growing up. "When I was sick, my grandmother would give me some herbal tea and say, 'This will make you feel better.'" Without the opportunity to work with Xiu-Min, TCM would never have entered Dr. Wang's professional life. Few people in the world have ever had the chance to study both disciplines in parallel. As far as I know, no one other than Dr. Li has had the precise scientific background and interest to delve into the mysteries of the immune system in this way, and no one else has had the combination of family and life circumstances that prepared them to take advantage of the geopolitical opportunities that have opened up in the past several decades. *Tianshi*, *dili*, *renhe*, indeed.

Dr. Li is very modest. She claims not to be an expert on all the disciplines that go into her work: "I am not a chemist, but I know enough about chemistry to direct the experiments." She is also not a statistician, but she knew enough about her own

相信,如果不是因为她个人独特的贡献,不是因为她在各种国家和国际委员会如此活跃地致力于发展补充和替代医学,西方医学和中医的结合将永远不会在这个国家甚至在世界上走这么远。

朱莉·王博士,李秀敏博士在西奈山的同事,也是那些委员会的成员,她是第二代华裔美国人,在美国出生长大,在美国一所医学院接受教育。她说她唯一和中医有接触是在她成长时:"我生病的时候,奶奶会给我一些草药茶,说喝了就好了。"如果不和秀敏搭档,中医不会成为王博士的研究方向。世界上很少有人同时学习这两种医学。据我所知,李秀敏博士所具备的有关免疫系统知识的精确科学背景和研究热情无人可比,并且,其他人也没有家庭和生活环境的结合以让其利用过去数十年开辟的地缘政治机会。李秀敏博士真是兼具了天时、地利、人和。

李秀敏博士非常谦虚。她说自己不是什么都懂:"我不是化学家,但我对化学的了解足以指导实验。"虽然她也不是统计学家,但她对自己在研究方面的抱负有足够的了解,所

ambitions in research to study statistics, one of the critical tools, in medical school.

When I was trying to make sense of Chinese medicine in books, I thus took her at her word that it wasn't necessary to study the *meridians*, one of the tenets of TCM physiology, or to know which diseases, medicines, and foods are considered hot and cold, or which ones rise from the spleen or descend from the liver. But it is not enough to know that these medicines work. As Dr. Li and one of her many coauthors have written, "It is insufficient to investigate the clinical efficacy of CAM (complementary and alternative medicine) without giving priority to elucidating the mechanistic actions of these therapies. In food-allergy research, as we struggle to define the roles of specific immune cells, portals for allergen sensitization, and the role of food allergy in setting the stage for more severe allergic diseases later in life, it is important to incorporate what we learn from CAM into this paradigm."[1]

There are no Chinese molecules and Western molecules. Says Dr. Sicherer: "The good news for science is that this is being done by pharmaceutical protocols. Just because something is natural and it works doesn't mean it can be safely used. Dr. Li's work starts with safety before effectiveness, even though she has this body of medicine from China to draw on, and studies animals before humans. She meets all regulatory and ethical requirements."

In effect, Dr. Li's work starts from proven

以她学习了统计学,这是医学(研究中)的一种重要工具。

当我学习中医时,我就想起她的话:没必要研究中医生理学理论之一的经络,或知道哪些疾病、药物和食物的寒热属性,或哪些病来源于肝脾。但仅仅知道药物起作用是不够的。李秀敏博士和她的一个合著者写道:"没有阐明这些疗法的机制就探讨补充和替代医学(CAM)的疗效是不够的。在食物过敏研究中,当我们努力确定特定免疫细胞的作用,过敏原致敏的途径,以及食物过敏在晚年为更严重的过敏疾病奠定基础方面的作用时,将我们从 CAM 中学到的知识纳入这一范式是很重要的。"

没有中国医学分子和西方医学分子之别。史可瑞博士说:"对于科学来说,好消息是现在的制药方案已经可以做到这一点。仅仅因为某些东西是天然的而且有效,并不意味着它可以安全使用。尽管李秀敏博士有中医知识可以利用,并且在做人体实验前做过动物实验,但李秀敏博士的工作仍然将安全放在效率之前。她的工作符合所有管理和道德要求。"

实际上,李秀敏博士的工作是从

---

① Julia A W, Xiu-Min L. Alternative and complementary treatment for food allergy[J]. Immunology and Allergy Clinics of North America, 2012, 32: 135-150.

treatment and works from the bottom up to show why it is safe and effective. She and coauthor Laverne Browne, PhD, described the rigor of proof this way: "Unlike synthetic drugs that begin with preclinical laboratory studies, botanical drug development from TCM has the advantage of long-term experience in human beings and generally an established safe profile. However, standardization of herbal formulas is challenging because the complex mixtures of herbs contain many constituents that have not been clearly defined. An essential requirement for clinical investigation of a botanical drug is an IND [investigational new drug] approval by the FDA [Title 21 Code of Federal Regulations 312.23 (a)]. The most unique section in this IND is the Chemical, Manufacturing, and Control (CMC) Data [21 CFR 312.23(a) (7)] requirement, which differs from that required for synthetic drugs. Given the unique characteristics of herbal mixtures, the FDA frequently relies on a combination of tests when the active chemicals are not well defined. HPLC [high-performance liquid chromatography] fingerprints, assays of characteristic markers, and biological assays are accepted methods to ensure quality, potency, and consistency of botanical drugs."①

What is the alternative from Western medicine? I read about the full spectrum of allergic diseases all the time and have somehow managed to enlist leading scientists and practitioners in writing for our website. Insights into the mechanisms of allergy are exploding.

有效的疗法开始的,从下到上展示为什么它是安全而有效的。她和合著者拉维恩·布朗博士以这种方式描述了严格的实验方法:"不同于从临床前实验室研究开始的合成药物,中医药的植物药开发具有人类长期经验的优势,而且总体上已确立了安全性。然而,中药方剂的标准化是有挑战性的,因为草药的复杂混合物含有许多未明确的成分。植物药的临床研究的基本要求是获得FDA[联邦法规第21号标准312.23(a)]的IND[研究性新药]批准。该IND中最独特的部分是化学、制造和控制(CMC)数据[21 CFR 312.23(a)(7)]要求,与合成药物所需要的不同。鉴于草药混合物的独特特性,当活性化学品未明确时,FDA经常依赖于组合测试。HPLC[高效液相色谱法]指纹图谱,特征标记物测定法和生物测定法是确保植物药物的质量、效力和一致性的公认方法。"

西医的替代方法是什么?我一直在阅读各种有关过敏性疾病的信息,并成功地为我们的网站招募了顶尖的科学家和医生。对过敏机制的了解正在激增。这里有很多好的科学文章,但不知何故,如标题为《抗

---

① Xiu-Min L, Laverne B. Efficacy and mechanisms of action of traditional Chinese medicines for treating asthma and allergy [J]. Journal of Allergy and Clinical Immunology, 2009, 123(2): 297 – 306.

There is a lot of good science, but somehow, articles with titles like "Anti-IL-5 Therapy Reduces Mast Cell and IL-9 Cell Numbers in Pediatric Patients with Eosinophilic Esophagitis [EoE]" don't point to anything like a broad-based "cure" in the foreseeable future. Even if a convenient way to synthesize anti-IL-5 agents and administer them to patients were found, it would be years before we knew whether it constituted an effective therapy for EoE, a potent and painful allergy of the digestive system, and at what cost. Synthetic antibodies to allergic effector cells are massively expensive.

The road from clinical insight to useful treatment is very slow. In 2012, I heard Dr. Arnold Levinson of the University of Pennsylvania challenge an audience of allergists to name a single real breakthrough in asthma treatment since the development of inhaled corticosteroids in 1944, which really only became economical with the discovery of the active ingredient *diosgenin* in wild Mexican yams in 1980.[①] No one raised a hand.

Standard allergy treatment is effective as far as it goes, but to a great extent, it just continues the stalemate treatment of the past hundred years, and for food allergy, it offers very little. With the rate of food allergies tripling over the past ten years, particularly peanut allergy, which is outgrown only 20% of the time, we face a crisis of accommodation in schools and restaurants, to name just two. Long term, institutions such as the military will be foreclosed to large numbers of otherwise qualified recruits, as Dr. Anna Nowak-

IL-5 治疗减少嗜酸性粒细胞性食管炎[EoE]儿童患者的肥大细胞和 IL-9 细胞数量》的文章没有指出任何在可预见的未来能广泛运用的"治愈方法"。即使发现了一个合成抗 IL-5 剂,并且可以把它们用在病人身上便捷的方法,我们也需要好几年的时间才能知道对于 EoE 这种强烈而痛苦的消化系统过敏来说它是不是一个有效的疗法,以及其代价是什么。另外,针对过敏效应细胞的合成抗体非常昂贵。

从临床观察到有效治疗道阻且长。2012 年,我听说宾夕法尼亚大学的阿诺德·莱文森博士挑战了台下一群过敏症专家,让他们说出自 1944 年以来治疗哮喘的吸入性糖皮质激素的真正的独一无二的突破。这只是一项实际上促进经济的发展,即 1980 年在墨西哥野生山药中发现了有效成分薯蓣皂苷元,但没有人举手。

标准过敏治疗是有效的,但在很大程度上,它只是继续过去几百年的僵化治疗,而对食物过敏提供的帮助很少。过去十年,食物过敏的发生率翻了三倍,尤其是花生过敏,在过去的几年中增长了 20%,我们面临着学校提供的食宿所带来的危险,这只是其中的两个问题。如西奈山的安娜·诺瓦卡·魏格森博士写的一样,

---

① http://en.wikipedia.org/wiki/Diosgenin.

Wegzryn of Mount Sinai has written.①

Many parents are taking matters into their own hands by forking over large sums to allergists who offer desensitization through OIT even though it is regarded as experimental and not FDA approved. I am sympathetic to these parents because OIT, although not a cure, does seem to offer limited protection against accidental ingestion for some people.

If a willingness to pay out of pocket for OIT is one measure of how anxious families are for relief from the day-to-day battle, so is their openness to alternative medicine. Large numbers of families have sought alternatives, although the numbers reported vary from one study to another. The 2002 National Health Information Survey showed that 36% of adults used CAM—"62% if prayer was included".② A 2006 survey③ of patients generally, not just for allergies, found that unproven or disproven diagnostic methods and (CAM) were used by approximately 20% of respondents, although they weren't impressed with the results. The survey also found that, given a choice, many would prefer herbal therapies to pharmaceutical drugs. By 2009, there were reports that 62% had used a CAM treatment and 26% had done so at the suggestion of a physician. Many of these responses undoubtedly included recommendations to use certain vitamins, which, like prayer, fall under the broad

长期以来像军队这样的机构拒收大量其他方面都合格（而有食物过敏史）的新兵。

许多家长为了解决问题，向提供 OIT 脱敏治疗的过敏症专科医生支付了一大笔钱，尽管 OIT 是实验性的，而不是 FDA 批准的。我对这些父母表示同情，因为 OIT 虽然不能治愈过敏，但对一些人来说似乎对意外摄入（过敏原）提供了有限的保护。

如果为 OIT 自付费用的意愿是衡量一个家庭为了摆脱日常战斗的焦虑程度的标准，那么也是衡量他们对替代医学的开放程度的一个标准。从一项研究到另一项研究，虽然报告的数字不同，但仍表明大量家庭已经转向替代医学。2002 年国民健康信息调查显示，36% 的成年人使用 CAM——如果包括祈祷则为 62%。2006 年的一项不仅仅是针对过敏患者的调查发现，有将近 20% 的调查对象使用了未经证实或不成熟的诊断方法和 CAM，尽管他们对结果并不满意。调查还发现，如果可以选择，许多人更喜欢草药疗法而不是药物。到 2009 年，有报告称，62% 的人使用 CAM 治疗，其中 26% 的人根据医生的建议这样做。毫无疑问，这些

---

① http://www.asthmaallergieschildren.com/2013/04/18/food-aller-gies-taking-the-long-view/.

② Renata J M E, Catherine M W, Philip J G, et al. Complementary and alternative medicine for the allergist-immunologist: where do I start? [J]. Journal of Allergy and Clinical Immunology, 2009, 123(2): 309-316.

③ Jimmy K, Jennifer I L, Anne M-F, et al. Use of complementary and alternative medicine by food-allergic patients[J]. Annals of Allergy, Asthma & Immunology, 2006, 97(3): 365-369.

heading of CAM. [1]

Patients seeking a path between mainstream and alternative medicine are often hamstrung by doctors' unwillingness to explore these options, however. Patients with allergic diseases are more likely to seek alternative treatments than those with any condition other than lower back pain. [2] As Dr. Renata J. M. Engler has written:

It has been easier to ignore the whole area of CAM as "placebo" or "not effective" and many patients complain that it is difficult to find a health care provider willing to partner with alternative practitioners or to monitor them if they choose an herbal or other CAM therapeutic trial outside the Food and Drug Administration-approved pharmaceutical industry. [3]

This does provide an opening for TCM, particularly as health-care costs have grown exponentially. As Dr. Li and Julia Ann Wisniewski, MD, one of her many collaborators, have written, "we have an obligation to our patients to understand their reasoning and interest in complementary treatments and to help them to make educated decisions about the potential risks and benefits of each. For patients with severe disease and limited conventional therapeutic options, or for those who have suffered from unwanted side effects of conventional

回应中有许多建议包括使用某些维生素,就像祈祷一样,属于 CAM 的广义范畴。

然而,寻求主流和替代医学之间路径的患者,常常受到医生不愿意探索这些选择的限制。比起除了腰痛以外的任何疾病,过敏性疾病患者更倾向于寻求替代治疗。正如勒娜特·J.M.恩格勒博士所写:

CAM 的整个领域更容易引起患者忽略,被当作"安慰剂"或"没有效果的",并且许多患者抱怨如果他们选择草药或其他在食品和药物管理局批准的制药业外的 CAM 治疗试验,很难找到愿意与替代医师合作或监督他们的医疗保健提供者。

这为中医提供了一个机会,特别是当医疗保健费用急剧增长时。李秀敏博士和茉莉娅·安·维希涅夫斯基(她众多合作者中的一个)写道:"我们有义务让我们的患者理解他们对补充治疗的想法和兴趣,并帮助他们对潜在风险和益处作出合理的决定。对于患有严重疾病和常规治疗选择有限的患者,或对于那些已经遭受常规治疗副作用的患者,我们

[1]　Mainardi T, Simi K, Bielory L. Complementary and alternative medicine: herbs, phytochemicals and vitamins and their immunologic effects[J]. Journal of Allergy and Clinical Immunology, 2009, 123(2): 283-294.

[2]　Leonard B. Complementary and alternative interventions in asthma, allergy, and immunology[J]. Annals of Allergy and Immunology, 2004, 93(2): S45-S54.

[3]　Renata J M E. Alternative and complementary medicine: a source of improved therapies for asthma? A challenge for redefining the specialty? [J]. Journal of Allergy and Clinical Immunology, 2000, 106(4): 627-629.

therapies, we should break the cultural and social barriers to accessing complementary therapies that have been proved to be safe and beneficial."①

Dr. Li's team turns ordinary mice into peanut-allergic mice by feeding them a combination of cholera toxin and crushed peanuts. Then they use herbal concoctions to reverse the process. They have completed their animal studies, and as you will read, are now in human trials.

This research is conducted in compliance with the standards set by the National Center for Complementary and Alternative Medicine (NCCAM) of the National Institute of Health (NIH). Although many critics contend that NCCAM began as cover for the supplement industry, successive legislation has made it a sponsor and watchdog for rigorous research such as Dr. Li's and may provide a pathway to market for effective treatment at a lower cost than standard pharmaceuticals. The record of NCCAM-supervised research has been more productive for what has been disproven than what has been proven. Dr. Craig Hopp, Program Officer, NCCAM, said in an email to me:

NCCAM-funded research in the natural products field has yielded limited data, if any, regarding products with "proven" efficacy. While we have seen some positive results regarding omega-3s, and hints of promise with other natural products in basic and pre-clinical research, to date, most of our large, randomized, placebo-controlled, clinical trials in this area, such as the Ginkgo Evaluation in Memory Study

应该打破文化和社会障碍,让他们获得已被证明是安全和有益的补充疗法。"

李秀敏博士的团队喂给普通小白鼠一种由霍乱毒素和碎花生构成的混合物,让它们对花生过敏。然后他们使用草药混合物来逆转过程。正如你所看到的,他们已经完成了动物研究,现在正进行人体试验。

本研究符合国家卫生研究所(NIH)国家补充和替代医学中心(NCCAM)制定的标准。虽然许多批评人士认为 NCCAM 最初是作为补充剂行业的掩护,但是连续的立法使其成为严格研究的帮助者和监督者,例如李秀敏博士的研究,并且可以提供一条以比标准药物更低的成本进入有效治疗的市场途径。NCCAM 项目官员克雷格·霍普博士在给我的一封电子邮件中说:

NCCAM 资助的天然产品领域的研究已经产生了关于具有"实证"功效的产品的有限数据(如果有的话)。虽然我们已经看到了一些关于 omega-3s 的阳性结果,以及在基础研究和临床前研究中与其他天然产物的希望的暗示,但是迄今为止,我们在该领域大部分的、随机排序的、安慰剂对照的临床试验,例如作为在记忆研

① Wisniewski and Li, op cit.

(http://nccam. nih. gov/research/results/gems), have not demonstrated greater efficacy versus placebo for the products, populations, and conditions studied.

As a nonscientist, I have struggled to understand the story of this research. I have slogged through dozens of peer-reviewed articles. When I started paying attention to medical literature a few years ago, I mentioned to a friend who is a public health authority and a department head at a major medical school that I read the abstracts and the discussion and couldn't make much sense of everything in between. He said, "That's all any of us do. " But for this project I did my best with the middle, too. There is a complex set of characters at work: not the scientists who did the work— this is not *The Double Helix*, which recounted the human drama behind the great discovery—but the many cells that comprise the immune system and the processes that regulate our health.

Although I deeply understand the impatience for a cure, I also have more respect and understanding for the rigors of the scientific method than ever before. Many mice have died, but human lives will be saved.

❷ The Parasite-Food Allergy Connection

Unlike asthma and other allergic diseases, food allergy is not described in the TCM literature.[①] When Dr. Li did her training in the 1970s and 1980s, it wasn't part of her curriculum. Even today, food allergies, particularly peanut allergy, are less common in China than in "industrialized" countries. By one account, the

究中的银杏评价(http://nccam. nih. gov/research/results/gems),对于所研究的产品、群体和条件,没有表现出比安慰剂更大的功效。

我不是科学家,但我一直在努力了解这项研究的详尽内容。我已经认真研读过几十篇同行评审的文章。当我几年前开始关注医学文献时,我向一位公共卫生当局的朋友兼一家大医学院的系主任提到,我读了摘要和讨论,却还是搞不明白。他说,"我们大家都是这样。"但对于这个项目,我也在中间尽了我最大的努力。工作中有一组复杂的角色:不是那些做这项工作的科学家——也不是讲述这一伟大发现背后的人类戏剧《双螺旋》——而是构成免疫系统的细胞和调节我们健康的过程。

虽然我深深地了解对于治愈方法的渴望,但是我也比以往任何时候更加尊重和理解科学方法的严谨性。虽然许多小鼠死了,但人类的生命会得救。

❷ 寄生虫与食物过敏的关系

与哮喘和其他过敏性疾病不同,中医药文献中没有食物过敏的描述。当李秀敏博士在20世纪七八十年代接受培训时,这并不是她课程的一部分。即使在今天,食物过敏,特别是花生过敏在中国也不像在"工业化"国家那么常见。据统计,即使人口总

① Xiu-Min L. Traditional Chinese herbal remedies for asthma and food allergy [J]. Journal of Allergy and Clinical Immunology, 2007, 120(1): 25－31.

raw numbers of peanut-allergic people in China are today estimated to be the same as in the United States, even though the population is four to five times as large. Roasting, the standard US cooking method, is thought to make peanuts more allergenic than boiling, frying, or pickling, which are more common elsewhere, because it leaves the allergens intact, whereas the other cooking methods partially denature them. [①]

TCM practitioners have been treating related diseases—allergic rhinitis, eczema, and asthma—for millennia with no clear idea of what the underlying mechanisms were, however; the antibody IgE was only identified in the late 1960s, by US researchers. When Xiu-Min came to New York from Johns Hopkins with Dr. Hugh Sampson to work at Mount Sinai, she established an outside clinic that would specialize in eczema. "People with bad eczema have a very low quality of life, and I thought that US medicine, which only treats the skin itself, wasn't adequate. If it's really bad, doctors do give oral prednisone, but that has side effects for the immune system overall."

"I had treated lots of eczema at the Chinese-Japanese Friendship Hospital in Beijing, where we treat it internally as well as topically, because there are different things that cause it. Even so, I was unprepared for the severity I saw. Dr. Sampson sent me two patients who were covered head to toe. There was no clear skin. It seemed to me that there were several different causes, so I had to prioritize and treat

数是美国的四到五倍,中国花生过敏人数的原始数据估算与美国是相同的。烘焙是标准的美国烹饪方法,被认为比在其他地区常用的煮、炸或腌制花生更易(诱发)过敏,然而烘焙留下的过敏原完整,而其他方法会使花生部分变性。

中医从业者已经治疗食物过敏相关疾病(过敏性鼻炎、湿疹和哮喘)上千年,但并不清楚其潜在机制是什么;抗体 IgE 在 20 世纪 60 年代末才被美国研究人员发现。当秀敏来到纽约,从约翰·霍普金斯大学再到跟着休·桑普森博士在西奈山工作时,她建立了一个专门针对湿疹的院外诊所。"患有湿疹的人的生活质量很低,我认为美国医学只治疗皮肤本身是不够的。如果湿疹真的很严重,医生确实会开口服泼尼松,但这对免疫系统有副作用。"

"我在北京的中日友好医院治疗了很多湿疹病人,我们进行内治和局部治疗,因为引起湿疹的原因各不相同。即使如此,我对于桑普森博士给我送来的两个从头到脚都是湿疹的病人的严重程度也没有准备。他们浑身没有清晰可见的皮肤。在我看来,有几个不同的原因,所以我不得不

---

① Lee J O, Lee J Y, Ahn Y H, et al. Ara h2 is not a major peanut allergen in Korea[J]. Journal of Allergy and Clinical Immunology, 2010, 125(2): AB225.

them all. The first thing was to bathe patients with herbal extracts, then use skin creams that were adapted from salves for treating wounds and burns, and when the skin started to show improvement, different skin creams and herbal tea could be used. "

The clinic practice built by word of mouth, and as the patient rolls grew, more and more patients presented with multiple food allergies, asthma, and sky-high IgE.

Back in the laboratory at Mount Sinai, food-allergy research focused on immunotherapy. Dr. Li says, "Dr. Sampson and I had been working on different kinds of peanut vaccine using animal models. In one study, we collaborated with Dr. Wesley Burks to investigate if a plasmid DNA *[①]-encod- ing Ara h2 gene therapy could prevent peanut anaphylaxis. Our idea was that if mouse host cells express Ara h2 gene and make Ara h2 protein, the immune cells may believe that Aha h2 is their own protein so that they would not react against it. "

Instead of inducing any protection, however, "We actually made the mice more prone to anaphylaxis. Normally, negative data would not be published, but we submitted our findings to *Journal of Immunology*, and the manuscript was accepted without revision. [②] We continued to collaborate with Dr. Burks and made engineered Ara h2 gene construct and then Ara h1 and 3 by modifying the Ara h1, 2, and 3 gene sequences.

按照轻重缓急来治疗。第一件事情是让患者用草药萃取物沐浴,然后使用从治疗伤口和烧伤的药膏改造而来的护肤霜,当患者皮肤开始慢慢改善,再使用不同的护肤霜和药茶。"

临床实践通过口口相传建立起来。随着病人的增加,出现越来越多的患有多种食物过敏、哮喘和极高含量的 IgE 的患者。

回到在西奈山的实验室,对食物过敏的研究主要集中在免疫疗法上。李秀敏博士说:"桑普森博士和我一直在使用动物模型对不同种类的花生疫苗进行研究。在一项研究中,我们与韦斯利·伯克斯博士研究质粒 DNA 编码——Ara h2 基因疗法是否可以预防花生过敏。我们的想法是,如果小鼠宿主细胞表达 Ara h2 基因,并且合成 Ara h2 蛋白,免疫细胞或许会相信 Ara h2 是它们自身的蛋白质,这样它们就不会对它产生反应。"

然而,(它)不但没有引起保护反应,"实际上,我们让小鼠更容易发生过敏反应了。一般情况下,负面数据是不会得到发表的,但是我们把发现提交给《免疫学杂志》后,我们的原稿没有作出任何修正就被接受了。我们继续与伯克斯博士合作,通过改造 Ara h1,2 和 3 的基因序列获得了 Ara h2 基因的结构,然后是 Ara h1 和 3 的

---

① ＊Genetic structure on a cell that can replicate independently of the chromosomes.
   细胞上的遗传结构能够单独复制染色体。

② Xiu-Min L, Chih-Kang H, Brian H S, et al. Strain-Dependent induction of allergic sensitization caused by peanut allergen DNA immunization in mice [J]. Journal of Immunology, 1999, 162(5): 3045 – 3052.

Our hypothesis was that the modified proteins would not be recognized by the IgE on the mast cells so that they would not cause reactions. We did see protection, but only partially, and only if the modified proteins mixed with heat-killed *Listeria monocytogenes* or *E-coli* bacteria as adjuvants. These immunotherapeutic approaches cannot be given orally; they require subcutaneous or rectal administration. Before I had the idea to test Chinese herbs, we had tested at least 10 different types of immunotherapy. "

The focus of her research changed when she sat with mothers of severely food-allergic children at a fundraising dinner. After Dr. Li described the excellent results she was getting with the herbal treatments for eczema, one of the mothers told Dr. Li about her daughter's food allergy and said she hoped Dr. Li could someday do the same with children like hers. After listening to this story and speeches by other mothers that were just as touching, Dr. Li says, "From that moment, I felt that as a physician-scientist, I had obligation to find a cure for these families. None of our tested immunotherapy was satisfactory in mouse models, which didn't hold out much promise for eventual human treatment. This is one of the reasons that I started to look for the potential of Chinese herbal medicines. "

Xiu-Min began studying the symptoms these mothers described, and something sounded familiar. She says, "I had memorized hundreds of formulas that used 500 different herbs. The connection with food allergies was blurry at first, but the symptoms began to sound like parasites. "

基因结构。我们的假设是肥大细胞上的 IgE 不识别被修正的蛋白质,所以它们不会发生反应。只要被修正的蛋白质与高温杀死的单核细胞增生李斯特菌或者与作为佐剂的大肠杆菌混合,我们就能看到抗过敏作用,但只对部分食物有效。这些免疫治疗方法没有口服药,它们需要皮下或直肠给药。在我有测试中草药的想法之前,我们测试了至少 10 种不同类型的免疫治疗。"

在一次筹款晚宴上,当李秀敏博士与患有严重食物过敏儿童的母亲坐在一起时,她的研究重点改变了。在李秀敏博士描述她用草药治疗湿疹得到的出色结果后,其中一个母亲告诉李秀敏博士她的女儿患有食物过敏,并说她希望李秀敏博士有一天同样可以治愈她女儿。在听完这个故事和其他母亲同样感人的话后,李秀敏博士说:"从那一刻起,我觉得作为一个医学研究者,我有义务为这些家庭找到治疗方法。我们测试的免疫疗法在小鼠模型中都不尽人意,这对最终的人类治疗没有多大希望。这是我开始寻找中草药潜力的原因之一。"

秀敏开始研究这些母亲描述的症状,她觉得有些听起来很熟悉。她说,"我记得数百种一共使用了 500 种不同草药的方剂。它们与食物过敏的联系起初是模糊的,但描述的症状开始听起来像寄生虫。"

She presented her ideas to Hugh Sampson, who told me, "At that point, I was interested in anything that might be used to treat food allergies." Unfamiliar with the Chinese tradition, he was skeptical but nevertheless gave the go-ahead with the condition that he would be active in the research at every stage.

Dr. Renata Engler is forthright in her appreciation of Sampson's decision. She says, "Given that there was nothing else new, Dr. Sampson's vision to pay attention to the long, anecdotal track record was precedent-breaking." As the work went on and started to show promise, Dr. Sampson worked with donors to direct more resources to it.

Intestinal parasites had played a key part in Dr. Li's early medical career. As a teenager, she had spent a couple of years in the mid-1970s in a farming village as a barefoot doctor, a job created in postrevolutionary China because medical care was so scarce, and the worms were a big part of her work. James Reston wrote in his 1971 article about his own experience with Chinese medicine: "Dr. William Chen, a senior surgeon of the United States Public Health Service [said] that before the Communists took over this country in 1949, four million people died every year from infectious and parasitic diseases and that 84 per cent of the population in the rural areas were incapable of paying for private medical care even when it was available from the 12,000 scientifically trained doctors."

Parasites are nasty. When they establish themselves in the intestines, they irritate or even perforate the

她向休·桑普森说了自己的想法,后者告诉我:"那时,我对任何可能用于治疗食物过敏的东西感兴趣。"由于不熟悉中国传统,休·桑普森对此持怀疑态度,但在每个阶段都可以积极参与研究的条件下,他还是同意了。

勒娜特·恩格勒博士直言对桑普森的决定的赞赏。她说,"鉴于当时没有什么新的东西,桑普森博士很有眼光,能够注意到久远的轶事记录(指中医文献中记载的),这是没有先例的。"随着工作的进行并开始显现希望,桑普森博士与捐助者合作,投入更多资源。

肠道寄生虫在李秀敏博士的早期医疗工作中发挥了关键作用。20世纪70年代中期,十几岁的她在农村当了几年赤脚医生,这是在"革命"后的中国创造出的一份工作,因为当时的医疗资源匮乏,而且寄生虫是她工作的主要部分。詹姆斯·雷斯顿在他1971年的文章中写到他自己对中医的检验:"美国公共卫生署高级外科医生威廉·陈博士说在1949年中国共产党建立新中国之前,每年有400万人死于传染病和寄生虫病,即使是有12 000名经过科学培训的医生可以提供医疗服务,84%的农村人口仍无法支付私人医疗费用。"

寄生虫很令人讨厌。它们在肠中定植时会刺激或甚至穿透肠壁,使

lining, leaving it vulnerable to penetration by large undigested molecules.

Formulas and Strategies, mentioned earlier, describes what happens:

Intermittent periumbilical (around the navel) pain… change in the complexion (usually wan, pale, or dark)… white spots in the malar (cheek) region, nighttime grinding of teeth, indeterminate gnawing hunger, vomiting of clear fluids…. If the condition is treated improperly and persists long-term, the patient will become emaciated and listless, lose interest in eating, and develop poor vision and hearing, dry hair, and a large distended abdomen. Infestation by parasites is a common cause of childhood nutritional impairment.

The life cycle of roundworms is as follows: Eggs pass through the stomach to the upper intestine, where they hatch into larvae. These burrow through the intestines, enter the bloodstream or lymphatic system, and end up in the lungs, where they mature. Nine days after ingestion, the time it takes for the larvae to pass from the lungs, up the airways, and into the mouth, they may be swallowed again and their life cycle repeated. The process from swallowing the eggs to having mature worms in the small intestine can take between two and three months, causing plenty of damage.

Parasites are nature's extortionists. Dangerous though they are, they are not ordinarily fatal. As with loan sharks and blackmailers, it is not in their interests from an evolutionary point of view to kill their hosts, just feed off them. Patients who survive an initial

其易于被未消化的大分子穿透。

前面提到的《方剂和疗法》详细描述了症状:

(肚脐周围)间歇性疼痛……肤色改变(通常苍白或晦暗)。(面颊)区域白斑,夜间磨牙,不定时的令人痛苦的饥饿感,呕吐清液……。如果治疗不当且病情长期持续,患者会变得消瘦,无精打采,食欲不振,进而发展为视力和听力差,头发干枯和腹部胀大。寄生虫侵染是儿童营养障碍的常见原因。

蛔虫的生命周期如下:卵通过胃到达肠的上部,在那里孵化成幼虫。幼虫穿过肠道,进入血液或淋巴系统,最终停在肺部并长大。虫卵被吞咽后的九天时间里,幼虫从肺部向上到呼吸道,再进入口腔,然后它们可能再次被吞咽,并且重复它们的生命周期。从吞咽卵到在小肠中成为成熟蛔虫的过程可能需要两至三个月,会严重损害人体。

寄生虫是大自然的敲诈者。尽管它们危险,但通常不致命。与放高利贷者和勒索者一样,杀死它们的宿主从进化的角度来看对它们没好处,所以它们只是取食于宿主。在初次

exposure have a defense in the form of IgE antibodies attached to their mast cells and basophils, which are on guard against re-exposure, or, in the case of most parasites, regeneration. ① Children are most at risk because their immune systems are too immature to get them through the initial exposure.

In contemplating the power of IgE as a weapon of food-allergy destruction, it helps to know how it works as nature intended it, as a defense against parasites, which can cause an increase in total serum IgE of 10 to 100 fold. ②

A study by Harvard researchers compared a group of "wild-type" mice to a control group that had been bred to be IgE deficient. As the name "wild-type" implies, these are mice that are held close to natural, not laboratory hybrids. They were all infected with *trichinella spiralis*, which causes trichinosis, known to chefs everywhere as the reason we don't serve rare pork. It kills about 50 people a year in the United States, usually from undercooked wild game as well as pork.

The wild-type animals mounted a robust IgE response that peaked on day 14 after primary infection, and the scientists concluded that "the role of IgE in immunity to *T. spiralis* is not restricted to facilitating the expulsion of adult worms from the intestine but also includes killing of larval stages of the parasite." ③

The authors of this study concluded that their

接触后患者具有附着于其肥大细胞和嗜碱性粒细胞的 IgE 抗体形式的防御,可防止再次接触,或对于大多数寄生虫是防止其再生。儿童最危险,因为他们的免疫系统太不成熟,不能幸免于最初的接触。

在考虑 IgE 作为破坏食物过敏的武器的力量时,有助于知道它如何出于本能防御寄生虫,这可以导致总血清 IgE 增加 10 至 100 倍。

哈佛研究人员的研究将一组"野生型"小鼠与已经培育为 IgE 缺陷的对照组进行比较。正如名称"野生型"所暗示的,这些是亲近自然而不是实验室杂交的小鼠。它们都感染了旋毛虫。旋毛虫可以引起旋毛虫病,这为各地大厨所熟知,也是我们要将猪肉煮熟的主要原因。在美国,每年约有 50 人死于这种疾病,通常感染于未煮熟的野味和猪肉。

野生动物作出了强有力的 IgE 反应,原发感染后第 14 天达到峰值,科学家们得出结论:"IgE 在旋毛虫免疫方面的作用不限于促进成虫从肠道排出,还包括杀死幼虫阶段的寄生虫。"

这项研究的作者总结说,他们的

① http://www.ehow.com/facts_5 5762 89_roundworms-life-cycle- humans. html.

② Nagaraji S, Raghavan R, Macaden R, et al. Intestinal parasitic infection and total serum IgE in a symtomatic adult males in an urban slum and efficacy of antiparasitic therapy[J]. Indian Journal of Medical Microbiology, 2004, 22(1): 55 – 56.

③ http://www.jimmunol.org/content/172/2/113.fiill.

work "provides support for the long-held but disputed notion that parasitic infections have provided the evolutionary pressure that has selected for the persistence of the IgE-Fc RI system." (Fc RI refers to the "high-affinity receptors" on effector cells to which IgE attaches while waiting for the antigens that will cause them to unleash the barrage of histamines and other mediators.)

In trying to visualize this mechanism in a food-allergic person, remember that intestinal worms are complex, multicelled animals, not a few isolated proteins. The immune response for such an intruder must be powerful and persistent. Now picture this same attack mobilized in response to a bite of a Reese's peanut butter cup.

TCM treatment for parasites augments natural defenses by paralyzing the worms and disrupting their reproductive cycle so they can be expelled before they can implant new larvae, while at the same time quelling destructive inflammation and relieving pain.

The chosen instrument of the initial effort was the nine-herb traditional formula *Wu Mei Wan* (WMW). According to Dr. Li, WMW was classically prescribed "for colic, vomiting, chronic diarrhea or dysentery, and collapse (also translated as syncope) caused by parasitic worms. WMW has also been recently reported to be effective for treating several other syndromes, such as drug-induced rash, neurogenic vomiting, asthma, chronic gastroenteritis, and colitis."[1]

工作"为长期存在但有争议的观点提供了证据,即寄生虫感染提供了进化压力,这种压力选择了持久的 IgE-Fc RI 系统。"(Fc RI 指的是 IgE 附着在效应细胞上的"高亲和力受体",在等待抗原释放出大量组胺和其他介质的时候,它们就会附着在这些细胞上。)

试图在一个食物过敏的人身上看到这一机制时,要记得肠道蠕虫是复杂的多细胞动物,不是几个孤立的蛋白质。对于这样的入侵者的免疫反应一定是强大而持久的。现在想象一下瑞茜咬了一口花生酱杯,同样的免疫反应发生了。

中医对寄生虫的治疗是通过麻痹蠕虫和破坏它们的生殖周期来增强自然防御能力,所以在它们植入新的幼虫前就可以把它们排出,同时消除破坏性炎症和缓解疼痛。

初次尝试所选择的方法是由九种中药组成的传统配方乌梅丸。据李秀敏博士说,乌梅丸传统上是治疗蛔虫所引起的"绞痛、呕吐、慢性腹泻或痢疾和厥证(也译作晕厥)的药。最近也有报道称乌梅丸在治疗其他症状上也是有效的,如药物性皮疹、神经性呕吐、哮喘、慢性胃肠炎、结肠炎。"

---

① Xiu-Min L. Traditional Chinese herbal remedies for asthma and food allergy [J]. Journal of Allergy and Clinical Immunology, 2007, 120: 25－31.

To the basic formula, two more ingredients particularly effective at immobilizing worms were added: *Zhi Fu Zi* (pharmaceutical name *Radix Lateralis Aconiti Carmichaeli Praeparata*) and wild *Ling Zhi* (*Ganoderma lucidum*, also known as *reishi* mushroom). (More about *Zhi Fu Zi* in a later chapter.) *Ling Zhi* of the quality Dr. Li wanted to use is rare and required using personal connections in China to locate a reliable supply in a remote, pristine region.

The new formulation was designated FAHF-1—short for Food-Allergy Herbal Formula-1.

Dr. Li told me that *Ling Zhi* has a special place in the TCM formulary and that it is mentioned in one of China's most treasured folktales, about a white snake that is turned into a beautiful woman. I asked a friend—the same one who gave me the proverb mentioned in chapter 1—about this story. He remarked that his father-in-law had played in the orchestra when the opera was performed at the Beijing Opera. He gave me a web link to a coherent retelling of the story where I found clues to the properties of the magic herb pertinent to treating food allergies.

Having been transformed from a white snake into Lady White, the newly formed woman meets a young man. They fall in love and marry. An abbot from a local temple, however, is on to her. During an annual festival devoted to driving away snakes, he urges this woman to take part in the ritual by drinking ritual *realgar* wine. She resists because she knows that it will turn her back into a snake, but she eventually agrees to

在基本的配方上，增加了两种特别有效的安蛔药成分：制附子（药品名称附子饮片）和野生灵芝（灵芝，又名赤芝）。（在后面的章节中会有更多关于"制附子"的内容。）李秀敏博士想用的这种品质的灵芝是罕见的，需要她利用在中国的人脉关系才能在偏远、原始的地区找到可靠的供应。

新配方被命名为 FAHF-1，即食物过敏中药方剂 1 的缩写。

李秀敏博士告诉我，在中医处方集当中灵芝的地位是特殊的，中国的一个民间传说中提到了灵芝，相传，一条白蛇变成了一个美丽的女人。现在我又向一个朋友询问了这个传说，就是我在第一章里提到过的告诉过我一个谚语的那个人。他说当（有关这个传说的）歌剧在北京上演时，他岳父曾在伴奏的管弦乐队里演奏。他给了我一个连贯性地讲述这个故事的网页链接，我发现这个传说中有与治疗食物过敏相关的魔法药草特性的线索。

从一条白蛇变成了白娘子，这个新生的女人遇到了一个年轻男人。他们坠入了爱河并结了婚。然而，当地一个寺庙的方丈却盯上了她。在一年一度的驱蛇节日里，这个方丈敦促白娘子参加仪式并且喝雄黄酒。她拒绝了，因为她知道，雄黄酒会把她变回蛇，但最后为了让她的丈夫高兴，她同意喝了，结果就有糟糕的事

drink to please her husband, with bad results. She passes out and reverts to a snake, whereupon her husband "dies" of shock. When she resumes her beautiful human form, she wakens, and seeing that her husband is dead, she declares, "I will fly to Kunlun Mountain and steal a miracle mushroom from the gods. That and nothing else can bring him back to life."

This being a fairy tale, there is a battle with enchanted animals guarding the mushroom, and other supernatural obstacles, but she secures a sample and returns home, where she feeds her husband a drink made from it. He is revived.

Still, although he is ignorant of events that took place while he was "dead," the husband is shaken, and it is only after a period of struggle that he and Lady White eventually live happily ever after.

Like many folktales, this story reveals truths about the world and society in which its creators lived, and observations about cause and effect that could be called scientific. It shows the centrality of parasites in community and personal health, and the value that people attached to treating them.

The part that really got to me, however, was the fact that the couple's lives are changed by the experience, and not for the better. The husband becomes tentative and fearful. This brush with death suggests anaphylactic shock, when the blood pressure plunges and the airways become constricted and fill with mucus. In autopsies, this is virtually

情发生了。她昏倒了，然后变回了蛇。于是，她的丈夫因为惊吓过度而死去。当她重新变回美丽的人形醒来后，看到她的丈夫死了。她发誓，"我要飞到昆仑山，从神仙那里偷到一个神奇的蘑菇。除了那之外，没有什么可以救活他"。

在这个传说当中，白娘子同守卫灵芝的神兽大战一场，但她还是成功拿到了一株灵芝，并返回家中。在家里，她给她丈夫喝了用灵芝做出的药水。她的丈夫复活了。

然而，她的丈夫还是有所动摇，尽管他对自己"死的"时候所发生的事一无所知，但在经过一段时间的挣扎之后，他和白娘子最终幸福地生活在一起。

像许多民间传说一样，这个故事揭示了造物主所生活的世界和社会的真相，以及可以被称为科学的因果观察。它揭示了寄生虫在群体和个人健康中的中心地位以及人们对治疗寄生虫病的重视。

然而，真正让我有所感触的是这对夫妇的生活被这段经历改变了的事实，并且是朝着不好的方向改变。之后，这个丈夫变得犹豫不决和害怕。与死神擦肩而过的经历导致了过敏性休克，血压突然下降、呼吸道收缩并且充满黏液。在尸检时，这实

indistinguishable from fatal asthma. ① The stamp of anaphylaxis on the lives of contemporary food-allergic families is indelible, particularly when the patient is a child.

As I have learned by communicating with many distraught mothers, once the threat of anaphylaxis enters the lives of families, the world changes. It becomes dark and ominous, and each casual ingestion of certain foods can be life threatening. The more I deal with food-allergic patients and particularly their mothers, the more I hear the echo of the tale of the white snake.

To a TCM practitioner also trained in Western science, as Dr. Li is, this is much more than a folktale about a folk cure. *Proving* the efficacy of classic formulas, *disproving* them (which is also part of science), and *improving* them is the focus of robust research in China. As Reston put it, "like everything else in China these days, it is on its way toward some different combination of the very old and the very new." I can't think of any more apt example of how very old and very new are being combined than in the promise that TCM holds for curing incurable diseases.

质上是不易被察觉的致命的哮喘。过敏反应给当下有食物过敏病人的家庭生活留下的印记是不可磨灭的，尤其当病人是一个孩子时。

我和许多心烦焦虑的母亲沟通后得知，一旦过敏反应威胁到她们的家庭生活，她们的世界就改变了，变得黑暗、危机重重。每一次偶然地摄入某些食物就会变成生命的威胁。我接触的食物过敏的病人越多，尤其是当接触到他们的母亲时，我就越多地想到《白蛇传》这个故事。

对于一个像李秀敏博士一样受过西方医学培训的中医来说，这不仅仅是一个有关于土方治病的传说。在中国，证明经方的疗效，证伪（这也是科学的一部分）并改良它们，这是中国人精确研究的重点。就像雷斯顿说的那样，"就像现在中国的其他东西一样，对很古老的和很现代的东西的一些不同的结合，中国有自己的方法。"有望新旧结合用于治疗疑难杂症，除了中医，我想不出任何更适当的例子了。

① Richard S H P, Ian S D R. Postmortem findings after fatal anaphylactic reactions[J]. Journal of Clinical Pathology, 2000, 53(4): 273 - 276.

PART TWO

The Science

These chapters primarily recount a series of painstaking experiments, starting with the creation of an animal model for testing, as well as explanations of other facets of the modern scientific method. They are followed by discussions of several newer lines of research that aren't complete yet but that indicate exciting new directions the science may take.

Until I made my way through the published articles, I had little appreciation for the conventions of scientific publishing, which involves recapitulating the background to the current experiment using the same or similar words and citations. To an amateur researching a particular area, they do appear to cover the same ground over and over again, often in the same or similar words, and cite the same references before getting to anything new. It's as if the Twelve Days of Christmas became the six months of Christmas and you had to sing every verse just to get to the next one. However, as Linda Miller (a PhD immunologist, a postdoctoral fellow at the National Cancer Institute, founding editor of *Nature Immunology*, and, incidentally, another cousin) explained to me that papers are written this way to both provide formal structure to thinking and facilitate experimental replication. Recapping the history in similar words and citations may be repetitious, but it provides

第二部分

科　学

本部分主要讲述了一系列艰苦的实验，从动物实验模型的建立开始，以及现代科学方法的其他方面的解释。接着是对一些较新研究路线的讨论，虽然不完整但却是科学可能采取的令人兴奋的新方向。

在我读完已发表的文章之前，我很不欣赏科学出版刊物的惯例，因为它们总是使用相同或类似的词汇和引文综述现行实验背景。对于研究某一特定领域的业余人士来说，这些科学家似乎只是一遍又一遍地研究同一内容，在得到新的研究成果前往往使用同样的话或类似的词语，引用也近乎相同。这就像为期十二天的圣诞节变成了六个月，而直到下一个圣诞节来临你必须唱每一首诗。然而，正如琳达·米勒（免疫学博士，美国国家癌症研究所的博士后，《自然免疫》的创刊编辑，也是另一个表亲）向我解释说，论文这样写是为了提供正式的思维模式和有效促进实验的可复制性。使用相似的词和引言确实显得累赘，但它提供了背景、

background, continuity, and context: "For replication, identical or similar experiments are initially performed to make sure your system is aligned with previously published work so that your new experiments proceed on a proven foundation."

Replicability is everything, one of the main principles of the scientific method, as my trusty Wikipedia reminds me. With all the scandals of the past several years about the quality of published research, I have begun to find this repetition reassuring, especially considering the pioneering nature of the work. Replicability lay at the heart of Dr. Sampson's determination to oversee the research with a skeptical eye. This was alien territory. It wasn't enough to show good data. He says, "I had the researchers repeat the experiments several times. The results were consistent; they utilized the appropriate science and hit all the standard immune markers."

Dr. Li's herbal formula is now the most advanced investigational drug in the history of the NCCAM. A great deal is riding on it, and the methods must be meticulous. The results of each study must not only satisfy the researchers but also their reviewers at the NIH.

Although I have done my best to clarify the literature, it is often tough sledding, full of obscure numbers and Greek letters. Sometimes it's hard to tell the interferons from the interleukins, and the T cells from the B cells, and so I thought it might be useful to have a preview of the chapters that follow.

连续性和语境:"为了保证可复制性,对于一致或相似的实验,要首先能确定你的体系是建立在先前发表的作品之上,这样新的实验才有足够坚实的基础。"

就像我所信赖的维基百科提示的那样,可复制性就是一切,是科学方法的基本原则之一。由于过去几年有关已发表成果的研究质量的丑闻,我逐渐发现这种重复令人心安,尤其是考虑到一些工作的前瞻性。桑普森博士持怀疑态度监督实验时,心里一直想着重复性。因为这是一个陌生的领域,仅仅展示良好的数据是不够的。他说:"有些研究人员重复实验数次。而结果是一致的,他们利用了适当的科学方法并标出了所有的标准免疫标记物。"

在美国补充替代医学国家中心的历史上,李秀敏博士的中药方是最先进的试验性新药。很多药物的发明是建立在中药之上的,当然方法必须严谨细致。每项研究的结果不仅要让研究人员满意,还要让美国国立卫生研究院的评审人员满意。

虽然我已经尽了最大努力来弄清楚文献,但这真不是一项简单的工作,满篇模糊的数字和希腊字母。有时很难区分干扰素和白细胞介素,T细胞和B细胞,所以我认为预览一下下面的章节可能会有帮助。

Establishing a Suitable Animal Substitute for People in Research

Obviously, you can't try this on human beings, and you can't wait around for lab animals to evolve the full set of deadly immune-system vulnerabilities as people. Mice are well established for this kind of research, but the challenge remained of inducing allergies using forced feeding of peanut extract with the help of a reagent to speed up the process, then determining whether the physiological responses were close enough to human responses to continue to use them in later work. Each time a new experiment commenced, it began with the same strain of mice and identical procedures.

A First Test of Efficacy—FAHF-1

FAHF-1 was a "beta version" of the food-allergy herbal formula. The classical version of WMW that constitutes the basis for this treatment contains ingredients that raise some regulatory red flags for use in humans but were adequate for testing in mice. Even in this version, the experiment showed that the drug could be administered safely, that it mitigated allergic symptoms, including the most serious (anaphylaxis), and that the biochemistry associated with these changes could be studied. Most important, here was convincing evidence that a Th1-Th2 imbalance might be correctible, that an allergic immune system could be "cured."

Process of Elimination

This chapter covers the thinking behind the regulatory concerns about a couple of the ingredients in the classic formula. The substitutions and recalibrations may surprise you.

为研究中的人寻求合适的动物替代品

显然,你不能用人类做实验,你也不能等着实验室动物进化出有着像人类一样的免疫系统。小鼠是公认的此类研究的实验对象,但在试剂的帮助下强制喂食花生提取物,然后观察它们生理反应上是否足够接近人类的反应,继而确定在后续研究中是否继续使用它们的过程中依然存在挑战。每次一个新的实验,都使用相同品系的小鼠和同样的步骤。

对食物过敏中药方剂 1 号 (FAHF-1) 的第一次疗效测试

FAHF-1 是食物过敏一个"测试版"的中药方剂。乌梅丸的传统配方构成此治疗的基础,虽然其含有的成分可能触及药品监管,但这些足以用来测试小鼠。实验表明,甚至这个版本中的药物也可以安全给药,可以减轻过敏症状,其中包括最严重的(过敏反应),并且可以研究与这些变化相关的生物化学。最重要的是,有令人信服的证据表明,Th1-Th2 失衡及过敏的免疫系统可以被"治愈"。

减药过程

本篇涵盖了对经方中一些成分加以监管背后问题的思考。替代效应和修正改良会让你大吃一惊。

Proof

This chapter recounts two experiments that not only demonstrate the efficacy of FAHF-2 on all key measures but also, for the first time, show that the curative effects last well past the cessation of therapy.

Whole Greater Than the Sum of Its Parts

When you start with an ancient formula arrived at through centuries of trial and error, you have to wonder if modern science might reveal some shortcuts. Maybe fewer herbs might yield the same results, which would make the whole process of gathering the ingredients, refining, and packaging that much simpler and cheaper. To that end, each of the ingredients was tested individually. The medicinal properties were studied, and it was revealed that in fact, the whole package was more effective than any lesser combination.

How Long Does It Last?

This chapter explores what amounts to a philosophical divide in food-allergy treatment as well as a medical one—the desirability and efficacy of oral immunotherapy for food allergies to desensitize them and raise the threshold of accidental ingestion on the one hand compared to lasting correction of the immune system on the other. The Mount Sinai teams show that "*In vivo* (in the live mice) and *in vitro* (in a laboratory culture) this was the first evidence that an herbal formula can produce complete, long-lasting protection against peanut-induced anaphylaxis."

Human Trials

Research doesn't follow a straight line. Before they were done with the mice, the Sinai team began to

验证

本篇讲述了两个实验,不仅证明了FAHF-2对所有关键指标的疗效,而且首次表明,该疗法的疗效可以持续到治疗结束后很久。

整体大于部分之和

当你从经过几个世纪的试验得来的方剂开始的时候,你一定会好奇现代科学是否可能提供一些捷径。也许更少的草药可能会产生相同的结果,这将使收集成分、精炼和包装的整个过程更简单、更便宜。为此,分别对每种成分进行了测试。对药物性能进行研究后发现,事实上,完整的配方比任何减药组方更有效。

持续多长时间?

本篇探讨了在食物过敏治疗和医学治疗方面的哲学分歧,一方面是使食物过敏脱敏并提高意外摄入的阈值,另一方面是对免疫系统的持续修正。西奈山团队表示"体内(在活小鼠)和体外(在实验室培养)是一个中药方剂对于减少花生过敏可以产生完整的长期保护的第一个证据。"

人体试验

研究不是一帆风顺的。在用老鼠做实验之前,西奈山的研究小组就

plan for the day when they could safely begin to work with people. This entailed thinking about what form, liquid or pills, would work best, and then showing whether, apart from efficacy, FAHF-2 could be administered without harming human subjects.

Too Many Pills

Even a "miracle cure" is useless if patients can't stand to take the medicine. In transforming WMW from a centuries-old herbal treatment into a 21st century medicine, the researchers had to consider Western tastes and customs. As anyone who has been told to continue a course of antibiotics even after starting to feel better knows, medication fatigue is a real thing. Brewing tea from a combination of herbs in quantity and drinking every day would be a burden for American mothers and kids. Pills are better— but how many?

Documenting the Quest for a Cure

Researchers must document annually all investigational drugs regarding how far they have come, where they plan to go, and how they intend to get there. This chapter provides the snapshot of progress taken in October 2012 showing how human subjects have reacted and describing procedures for the next phase of trials.

❸ Establishing a Suitable Animal Substitute for People in Research

In 1945, writer E. B. White published the classic children's novel *Stuart Little*, in which a New York woman gives birth to a very unusual child—a mouse with the intellect and feelings of a human being. White was prescient. Genomics research has revealed to us

已经开始计划哪一天他们可以安全地开展人类试验了。这需要考虑以哪种形式进行会最有效，液体还是药片，而且除了证明功效，还要证明FAHF-2 可以在不伤害人类受试者的情况下使用。

药丸数量太多

如果病人不能忍受服药，即使是"灵丹妙药"也无济于事。在将乌梅丸从一种古老的草药疗法转变为21世纪的医学时，研究人员不得不考虑西方人的口味和习惯。即使感到好转的人在得知要继续服用抗生素时，都会体会到药物疲劳是真实存在的。对美国的母亲和孩子们来说，每天冲泡大量的草药并饮用将是一种负担。药丸是更好的——但要吃多少呢？

记录对治愈方法的探索

研究人员必须每年记录下所有试验性新药，包括他们取得了多大进展、计划取得什么样的进展以及打算如何达到目标。本篇概述了在2012年10月所取得的进展、人类受试者的反应并描述下一阶段的试验程序。

❸ 为研究中的人寻求合适的动物替代品

1945 年作家 E.B. 怀特出版了经典儿童小说《精灵鼠小弟》，讲述了一个纽约女人生了一个非常不寻常的孩子——一个有着人类的智力和情感的老鼠。怀特是有先见之明

that mice and humans have considerable genetic overlap. According to a 2010 European Commission paper, "99% of human genes are conserved in mice." Although other animals—dogs, pigs and primates, particularly—have even more in common with people than mice do, this same paper pointed out, "Working with these large animals is extremely expensive and is fraught with ethical concerns"—not to mention the logistical nightmare of transporting large numbers of them to the 17th floor of the Annenberg Pavilion at Mount Sinai. The small size and short generation times of mice, ease of breeding and keeping, and decades of their use in research have given scientists detailed understanding of mouse biology and genetics. ①

Despite long use of TCM compounds with human patients, the researchers at Mount Sinai had to demonstrate the safety and efficacy of those compounds in animals according to exacting protocols. Whether applying to the NIH or the Department of Defense (DOD), which sponsor most basic research, these are your tax dollars at work. Dr. Li says regulators don't want too much novelty. Writing grant proposals and gaining scarce funding is an orderly process, and the NIH shies away from research that involves too great a leap; likewise, peer-reviewed journals. The closer a project gets to market, the larger the share of support must be gathered from nongovernmental sources.

的。基因组学的研究向我们揭示,小鼠和人类有相当大的遗传重叠。根据2010年欧盟委员会的一份文件,小鼠拥有99%的人类基因。虽然其他动物如狗、猪,特别是灵长类动物比起小鼠与人有更多共同处,但文件同时指出拿这些大型动物做研究是非常昂贵的,并且充满了伦理问题,更不用说把它们大量运到西奈山安纳伯格馆的17楼,这简直就是噩梦。小鼠的体积小,繁衍时间短,易于繁殖和饲养,并且在几十年的研究中,科学家们已详细了解了小鼠的生物学和遗传学规律。

尽管人类患者已经长期使用中药混合物,但西奈山的研究人员必须根据严格的规程证明这些化合物在动物身上的安全性和有效性。是否向支持最基本研究的机构如美国国立卫生研究院或国防部申请,这些是必须要做的。李秀敏博士说,监管机构不希望有太多的新鲜事物。撰写资助提案和获取有限的资金是一个有序的过程,并且美国国立卫生研究院要避开涉及太大跨度的研究,同样评审期刊也是如此。一个项目越接近市场,来自非政府组织的支持就越大。

---

① http://ec.europa.eu/research/health/pdf/summary-report-25082010_en.pdf.

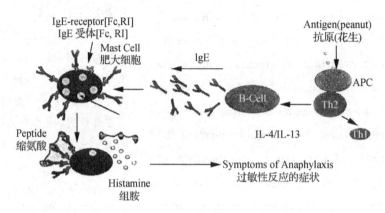

Immunopathogenesis of Food Allergy
食物过敏免疫发病机理

Regulators—and malpractice lawyers—want a good paper trail. As Renata Engler and colleagues put it："Ultimately, the standard of care will be determined by expert witness testimony in a court of law and is the same for all physicians regardless of whether they use conventional or CAM therapy."[1]

Fair enough. Peanut allergies are too dangerous to subject human beings to a systematic program of food challenges before, during, and after treatment. Even minute amounts of allergen can be fatal, and placebo-controlled trials could be catastrophic. Furthermore, although the allergy epidemic developed through thousands of seemingly random changes in the human immune system over decades, for research, that process had to be compressed into weeks in the lives of test animals.

Thus commenced in 1999 an effort to generate a *murine* model of peanut-induced anaphylaxis—that is, a rodent model, not the stuff you put in sore eyes.[2]

监管部门和负责医疗事故的律师想要一个完美的文件档案。正如勒娜特·恩格勒和她的同事所言："最终，护理的标准将由鉴定专家在法院决定，对所有医生来说都是一样的，不论其是否使用传统或 CAM 疗法。"

这是有道理的。花生过敏是非常危险的，在治疗前、治疗中、治疗后，都不能对人类进行系统性的食物过敏测试。即使少量的过敏原也可以是致命的，安慰剂对照试验可能是灾难性的。此外，尽管几十年来人类免疫系统中数千个看似随机的变化导致了过敏病流行，但为了研究，这个过程必须压缩到实验动物几个星期的生命期。

因此，于 1999 年开始努力创造一个花生引起的过敏反应小鼠模型——啮齿动物模型，而不是直接放

---

① Engler, With, Gregory, Jellin, op cit. p. 312.

② Xiu-Min L, Denise S, Soo-Young L, et al. A murine model of peanut anaphylaxis：T- and b-cell responses to a major peanut allergen mimic human responses[J]. Journal of Allergy and Clinical Immunology, 2000, 106(1)：150-158.

There had previously been no completely suitable animal model of peanut allergy to test the efficacy and safety of immunologic therapies.

The standard shortcut, *intraperitoneal* sensitization —direct injection of highly allergenic peanut proteins into the thin, or *serous*, membrane lining the walls of the abdominal and pelvic cavities—was no good. If you're going to model food allergy, it's better to come as close to actual eating as possible. The vision was for an accessible, ingestible botanical treatment, as opposed to a high-priced hospital treatment, with stomach tissue as permeable to the allergens as with naturally occurring food allergies. The alternative chosen was *intragastric* administration—force-feeding doses of peanut antigen and adjuvant.

Tools of the Trade

First, a call went out to the Jackson Laboratory, a publicly supported national repository for mouse models in Bar Harbor, Maine, that was established in 1929. This nonprofit center pioneered the use of inbred laboratory mice to uncover the genetic basis of human development and disease, and today is the site of original research in areas that include cancer, development and aging, immune system and blood disorders, neurological and sensory disorders, and metabolic diseases as well as being the supplier of mice for other laboratories. In 2002, the lab supplied approximately two million mice to the international scientific community.

The process of creating peanut allergy in mice began with an order for five-week-old mice of strain C3H/HeJ, described in the Jackson catalogue as "a

进入类疼痛的眼睛。此前一直没有完全适合花生过敏的动物模型来试验免疫疗法的安全性和有效性。

标准的捷径是腹腔内致敏——将高致敏性花生蛋白直接注入连接腹腔和骨盆腔的薄壁或浆液膜——是没有什么用处的。如果你要模拟食物过敏,最好是尽可能地接近实际的饮食。这个构想是为了获得可以接受的可摄入植物性治疗,而不是高昂的医院治疗,胃组织对过敏原与天然存在的食物过敏一样都是可渗透的。替代选择是灌胃给药——强制喂食一定剂量的花生抗原和辅助剂。

交易工具

首先,一个电话打到了杰克逊实验室,这是一个公立的国家小鼠模型储存库,位于缅因州的巴尔港,成立于1929年。这个非营利性中心率先使用近亲交配的实验室小鼠来揭示人类发展和疾病的遗传基础,如今是癌症、发育和衰老、免疫系统和血液疾病、神经和感官障碍以及代谢性疾病等领域的原始研究地点,同时也是其他实验室小鼠的供应商。2002年,该实验室向国际科学界提供了大约200万只小鼠。

制造花生过敏小鼠的过程始于一份五周大的C3H/HeJ菌株的订单,C3H/HeJ菌株在杰克逊实验室

general purpose strain in a wide variety of research areas including cancer, immunology, and inflammation, sensorineural, and cardiovascular biology. "[1]

Crude extracts of the protein components Ara h1 and Ara h2, which are associated with the most serious allergic reactions more frequently than other components, were created from freshly ground whole peanuts. Cholera toxin was employed as an adjuvant to accelerate the development of allergies—not a small consideration, given the less-than-two-year lifespan of the typical laboratory mouse. Unlike many other bacteria, cholera toxin can resist the highly acidic environment in the stomach. When it arrives in the small intestine, it makes flagella, fibers, that rotate and propel the bacteria corkscrew-like through the mucus of the small intestine. [2][3] Furthermore, a component of cholera toxin has been shown to augment the degranulation of mast cells. [4]

In tiny concentrations, the toxin makes the tissues more permeable without actually causing cholera or otherwise damaging them. [5] Without this boost, the mucus would perform its normal job of protecting the tissue and would dilute the strength of the peanut allergen. Using the toxin helps bind antigens more

目录中被描述为"一种用于广泛研究领域的通用菌株,包括癌症、免疫学、炎症、感觉神经和心血管生物学。"

从新鲜花生中提取出来的蛋白质成分 Ara h1 和 Ara h2 的粗提取物,比其他成分更容易导致最严重的过敏反应。霍乱毒素作为一种辅助剂加速了过敏的发展,由于典型的实验室小鼠的寿命不到两年,这不是一个可忽略不计的因素。不同于其他所有细菌,霍乱毒素能抵抗胃部的高度酸性环境。当它到达小肠,它产生的鞭毛和纤维,旋转推动细菌螺旋似的通过小肠的黏液。此外,霍乱毒素成分已被证明能增加肥大细胞脱粒。

在低浓度下,毒素会使组织更易被渗透,而实际上不会引起霍乱或其他损害。如果没有这种刺激,黏液会发挥其正常的保护组织的作用,会削弱花生过敏原的强度。使用该毒素有助于把抗原与消化系统的组织更

---

[1] http://jaxmice.jax.org/strain/000659.html.

[2] A comparable process takes place in the airways in environments with high levels of air-borne "black carbon" from diesel fuels, among other things. The particles penetrate the mucus, allowing exposure to allergens and other irritants, inducing asthma that can be passed on to offspring (http://www.medscape.com/viewarticle/779819).
就好比在柴油燃料黑炭含量高的气管里发生的一种过程。颗粒物穿过黏膜,使得黏膜接触到过敏原和其他致敏物,引起像哮喘这种能传给后代的疾病(http://www.medscape.com/viewarticle/779819)。

[3] http://en.wikipedia.org/wiki/Cholera.

[4] Fang Y, Larsson L, Mattsson J, et al. Mast cells contribute to the mucosal adjuvant effect of CTA1-DD after IgG-complex formation[J]. Journal of Immunology, 2010, 185(5): 2935 − 2941.

[5] Joaquin S, Jan H. Cholera toxin: a friend & foe[J]. Indian Journal of Medical Research, 2011, 133(2): 153 − 163.

tightly to the tissue of the digestive system, where they can essentially bombard the T cells, triggering an immune response disproportionate to the threat. Dr. Li speculates that the strength of the allergic response is a function of the confusion of the innate immune system, which reacts to foreign invaders but lacks memory, and the adaptive system, which has the capacity to learn. As the IgE-equipped mast cells confront the allergens and degranulate, they release histamine and other mediators. Other cells that normally would not be involved in the allergic response perceive a growing emergency and send in " reinforcements. " Think of this as Air Force radar confusing a flock of geese with a squadron of enemy airplanes.

A group of mice were left naïve (i. e. , with no intervention) to serve as a control. In addition, mice in another control group were fed only the cholera toxin without the peanut antigen. These were " sham-sensitized " mice, which serve as an additional experimental control to ensure that the cholera toxin in the absence of peanut protein did not cause adverse effects in the mice compared to the untreated control. The experimental group was dosed with both cholera toxin and peanut extract.

Each mouse was fed with either 5 mg (equivalent to 1 mg of peanut protein; low dose) or 25 mg (equivalent to 5 mg of peanut protein; high dose) of ground whole peanut together with 10 micrograms of cholera toxin on day one with the initial dose and again on day 7. The low-dose-high-dose experiment was based on an established principle of immunology research, that low doses produce sensitization and high doses produce tolerance. Although the team strongly

紧密地结合起来,在消化系统中,抗原可以攻击 T 细胞,引发与威胁不相称的免疫反应。李秀敏博士推测,过敏性反应的强度是先天免疫系统和适应性系统混乱的结果,前者会对外来入侵者作出反应但缺乏记忆,而后者有学习能力。当配备 IgE 的肥大细胞对抗过敏原并脱粒时,能释放组胺等介质。在察觉到越来越多的紧急情况时,通常不参与过敏反应的其他细胞会派送"增援部队"。可以把这想象为空军雷达把一群鹅与一个中队的敌机混淆了。

一群没有受干预的小鼠作为一个对照组。此外,另一个对照组的小鼠只喂养霍乱毒素而没有花生抗原。这些是"假致敏"小鼠,作为一个额外的实验对照组,以确保在没有花生蛋白的情况下,与未经处理的对照组小鼠相比,霍乱毒素没有造成不利影响。实验组小鼠被喂了霍乱毒素和花生提取物。

第一天,喂食每只小鼠 5 毫克(相当于 1 毫克的花生蛋白;低剂量)或 25 毫克(相当于 5 毫克的花生蛋白;高剂量)磨碎的花生及 10 微克的霍乱毒素,第七天以同样剂量喂食。低剂量高剂量实验是基于免疫学研究的一个既定原则,即低剂量产生致敏性,高剂量产生耐受性。虽然

suspected this dosing strategy would produce the usual results, proving its validity in each particular experiment is part of the protocol.

Three weeks after the initial sensitization, mice were left unfed overnight. The next day, each mouse was challenged intragastrically by having pumped into its stomach 10 mg of crude peanut extract divided into two doses at 30- to 40-minute intervals. Mice surviving the first challenge; were rechallenged at week 5. Sham-sensitized mice and naïve mice were challenged in the same manner.

Measuring the Antibodies

Each week, and again one day before challenges, serum samples were drawn from each group of mice after feeding. These samples showed that peanut-specific IgE concentrations increased significantly from week 1 through week 5 in mice sensitized with low-dose peanut (5 mg per mouse) and cholera toxin and from week 2 through week 5 in mice sensitized with high-dose peanut (25 mg per mouse) as well as the toxin; however, levels were significantly higher in the low-dose group than in the high-dose group at both week 3 and week 5, as anticipated.

The First Challenge

Allergen-specific IgE antibodies are not the true measure of allergy. If they were, food allergies could be diagnosed by the numbers. One of the things that makes food allergies so vexing, however, is that an individual may have fairly substantial IgE levels and still not have a clinical allergy. Even the addition of a skin-prick test (SPT), in which a small amount of the offending food is introduced where it may or may not

该小组强烈怀疑这种给药策略会产生常见的结果,但在每一个特定的实验中证明其有效性是方案的一部分。

初次致敏后三周,小鼠整夜不予喂食。第二天,每只小鼠进行10毫克花生粗提取物的灌胃试验,分两次进行,间隔30到40分钟。在第一次刺激中存活的小鼠,在第5周再次进行刺激。假致敏小鼠和未处理组小鼠以同样的方式接受试验。

测定抗体

对每组喂食后小鼠每周提取一次血清样本,并且在刺激前一天进行第二次。这些样本表明,在那些一至五周用小剂量花生(每只小鼠5毫克)和霍乱毒素致敏的小鼠以及从二至五周用高剂量花生(每只小鼠25毫克)和霍乱毒素致敏的小鼠中,花生特异性IgE浓度明显增加。和预期一样,在第3周和第5周低剂量组的花生特异性IgE水平显著高于高剂量组。

第一次刺激

过敏原特异性IgE抗体不是过敏的真实衡量标准。否则,食物过敏可以通过数值得到诊断。然而,食物过敏让人烦恼的一点就是一些人有相当高的IgE水平却没有临床过敏反应。即使增加皮肤点刺试验(SPT),也并非是完全可靠的,因为在少量有害的食物被引入皮肤,这些食物可能与真皮层的肥大细胞发生反应,也可

react with the mast cells of the dermis, is not entirely reliable. Short of an oral food challenge, which is not a great screening tool because it may result in a severe reaction, the best allergists rely on an extensive history, which may lead to a diagnosis.

With mice, however, the scruples about inducing anaphylaxis do not apply, so three weeks after the initial sensitization, mice were fed with crude peanut extract at 30- to 40-minute intervals, and the scientists watched.

Within 10 to 15 minutes after the first dose, systemic anaphylactic symptoms started to emerge. The initial symptoms consisted primarily of visible reactions such as puffiness around the eyes and mouth, diarrhea, or both, followed by respiratory reactions, such as wheezing and labored respiration. The most severe reactions were loss of consciousness and death. As expected, the low-dose mice exhibited more severe reactions than those sensitized with the high dose. Fatal or near-fatal anaphylaxis occurred in 12.5% of low-dose-sensitized mice but in none of the high-dose mice. Sham-sensitized—those that received only the cholera toxin and not the peanut—and naïve mice did not show any symptoms of anaphylaxis.

The first measure was observation of "Type 1 hypersensitivity" scored on this scale:

0—no symptoms

1—scratching and rubbing around the nose and head

2—puffiness around the eyes and mouth, pilar erecti (hair standing on end), diarrhea, and reduced activity or standing still with an increased respiratory rate

3—wheezing, labored respiration, and cyanosis

能不发生反应。缺少的口服食物刺激并不是一种有效的筛选工具,因为其可能引起严重的不良反应。最好的过敏医师主要依赖可以指向明确诊断的广泛病史。

然而,并不用顾虑小鼠会被诱发过敏反应,所以在最初致敏三周后,每隔30到40分钟喂食小鼠粗制的花生提取物,其间科学家们进行观察。

喂食第一剂后10到15分钟,小鼠开始出现全身过敏症状。最初的症状主要包括眼睛和嘴巴周围的浮肿,腹泻,或者两者都有,其次是呼吸道反应,如气喘和呼吸困难。最严重的反应是意识丧失和死亡。正如预期的那样,低剂量组的小鼠表现出的反应比那些高剂量致敏组的更严重。在低剂量组的致敏小鼠中有12.5%发生致死或接近致命的过敏反应,而在高剂量的小鼠中则没有。那些只接受霍乱毒素而不是花生的假致敏的老鼠以及未处理组小鼠没有表现出任何过敏反应症状。

第一项措施是对"1型超敏反应"以下面量表进行评分的观察:

0——无症状

1——抓挠和摩擦鼻子周围和头部

2——眼睛和嘴巴周围浮肿,毛发持续性直立,腹泻,活动减少或呼吸频率增加时站立不动

3——喘息、呼吸困难、口周围紫

(blue coloring from loss of oxygen) around the mouth

4—symptoms as in number 3 with loss of consciousness, tremors, and/or convulsion

5—death

The Second Challenge

Two weeks later, the surviving mice were challenged again, resulting in more systemic anaphylactic reactions in both low- and high-dose mice.

One additional finding: A preliminary study had shown no significant anaphylactic reactions if mice were challenged only at week 5; thus, the challenge at week 3 appears to have served as an additional boosting dose. As in the week 3 challenge, symptom scores at the week 5 rechallenge were also significantly higher in the low-dose group than in the high-dose group. The 5-mg-per-mouse dose became the standard for all subsequent studies.

Test Tube Results Confirm Systemic Peanut Allergy and Anaphylaxis Similar to Humans

Skeptics will say quite rightly that people are not the same as animals, the 99% genomic profile notwithstanding. With allergies, however, the mechanisms of a response are quite well understood, and the processes that take place in both species are so similar that direct comparisons can be made both in observation and under the microscope. To understand how comparable they are, a brief look at how allergies happen is in order.

The weapons that our immune systems use to fight certain invaders such as allergens and parasites are housed primarily in effector cells called mast cells and basophils, as mentioned in the first chapter. Antigen-

绀(缺氧而呈青色)

4——症状同3,伴随意识丧失,全身震颤及/或抽搐

5——死亡

第二次刺激

两周后,对存活的小鼠再次进行刺激,更多的低剂量和高剂量组小鼠出现了全身过敏性反应。

此外还发现:初步研究表明如果小鼠只在第5周接受刺激则无明显过敏反应;因此,第3周的刺激似乎起到了额外的助推剂量作用。在第3周进行刺激后,在5周时高剂量组症状评分显著高于低剂量组。每只小鼠5mg的剂量已成为所有后续研究的标准。

试管结果证实全身性花生过敏和过敏反应与人类相似

怀疑者马上会说人和动物不一样,尽管有99%的基因组谱相同。然而,过敏的反应机制很好理解,并且发生过程在这两个物种间非常相似,可以直接观察,并在显微镜下直接比较。为了了解它们之间的可比性,我们来看看过敏发生的过程。

如第一章中提到的,在对抗如过敏原和寄生虫等入侵者时,我们的免疫系统使用的武器是效应细胞中的肥大细胞和嗜碱性粒细胞。抗原特

specific IgE attaches itself to high-affinity receptors on the effector cells: mast cells, which mostly lodge in tissues, although some circulate in the blood, and basophils, which only circulate. Mast cells are responsible for the early phases of an allergic reaction because they are present at the site of an exposure, whereas basophils, which take their time getting to the site, account for the late phases, and also encounter allergens that have found their way to other parts of the body. With, say, seasonal allergies, symptoms are generally confined to the area where the allergen is encountered, the sinuses. Part of the inflammatory response is for tissues to swell up and isolate the intense activity. Food allergens present themselves to numerous tissues as they pass from mouth to intestines, however, thus the multiplicity of symptoms, including oral itching and hiving, choking, and diarrhea and vomiting, as well as late-stage symptoms as stray proteins make their way through the blood.

The IgE antibodies look something like lobster claws sticking out from the effector cells and work in pairs. The allergens fit between the claws, forming a bridge, and when they do, the allergic attack begins. The mast cell *degranulates*; that is, it swells up and bursts, and *mediators* are released. When the mast cell's work is done, it's like a pinata after children have pounded it with sticks and all the toys and candy have been unwrapped. The state of the mast cells in the mice and the levels of certain chemicals in the blood would be a telling indicator of how allergic the mice actually were.

Sure enough, the percentage of degranulated mast cells found in the mice's ear tissue was significantly

异性 IgE 附着于效应细胞上的高亲和力受体：肥大细胞，主要存在于组织中，有些在血液循环中，而嗜碱性粒细胞仅存在于循环中。因为肥大细胞存在于与过敏原直接接触的地方，它们主要作用于过敏反应的早期阶段，而嗜碱性粒细胞需要花时间到达且主要作用于后期阶段，还会遇见到达身体其他部位的过敏原。此外，季节性过敏的症状通常局限于遇到过敏原的区域，即鼻窦。炎症反应的部分症状是组织肿胀和孤立的激烈活动。当食物过敏原从口腔进入肠道时会出现在许多组织上，因此会出现多种症状，包括口腔发痒、窒息、腹泻和呕吐，以及晚期游离态蛋白质通过血液而出现的症状。

IgE 抗体看起来像龙虾爪子一样从效应细胞中伸出并成对工作。过敏原会在爪子之间形成桥梁，当它们形成桥梁时，过敏反应就开始了。肥大细胞脱粒，即膨胀和破裂，并且释放炎症介质。当肥大细胞的工作完成了，就像孩子们用棍子敲打开了彩陶罐，可以看到所有玩具和糖果。小鼠体内肥大细胞的状态和血液中某些化学物质的含量，将是小鼠过敏程度的一个指标。

果然，花生致敏小鼠的耳组织肥大细胞脱粒百分率比对照组小鼠显

greater in peanut-sensitized mice than in control mice. Plasma histamine levels *[1] were also significantly higher in peanut-sensitized mice than in both sham-sensitized and naïve mice. An additional procedure called a passive cutaneous anaphylaxis (PCA) test was done, in which serum from the blood of one mouse is injected into the skin of another before the antigen challenge. This was done to rule out IgGl-mediated anaphylaxis, in which effector cells are activated through a receptor called Fc RIII and can be detected by different biomarkers than IgE reactions. Injection of sera from mice with peanut-allergy-induced reactions elicited a positive PCA reaction following the cutaneous injection of peanut extract, whereas injection of sera from normal wild-type mice did not cause any reaction.

In each additional test of T cells, B cells, and various measures of IgE binding, the ways mice responded to allergens in this model resembled human reactions.

Mission accomplished. The researchers had generated a murine model of peanut anaphylaxis. As with humans, these symptoms involved multiple target organs, including the skin, gastrointestinal tract, and respiratory system, with the most severe reactions being fatal. The way was cleared to induce peanut allergy in more mice, measure their reactions in greater detail, and finally, the researchers hoped, test for a cure.

著增加。花生致敏小鼠的血浆组胺水平也明显高于假致敏和未处理的小鼠。进行了附加的被动皮肤过敏反应(PCA)测试,即将一只小鼠的血清注射到另一只在抗原试验之前的小鼠体内。这样做是为了排除 IgG1 介导过敏,其中效应细胞通过 Fc RIII 受体激活效应细胞,可以通过不同的生物标志物而不是 IgE 反应检测。注射了花生过敏反应诱导小鼠的血清后的小鼠,在皮肤注射花生提取物后引起了阳性被动皮肤过敏反应,而注射正常野生型小鼠血清没有引起任何反应。

在每一个关于 T 细胞、B 细胞的额外测试中,以及对 IgE 结合的各种测量中,小鼠对该模型过敏原的反应方式类似于人类反应。

任务完成了。研究人员已经建立了花生过敏的小鼠模型。对于人类来说,这些症状涉及多个目标器官,包括皮肤、胃肠道和呼吸系统,最严重的反应是致命的。研究人员为在更多的小鼠身上诱发花生过敏扫清了道路,并对它们的反应进行了更详细的测量,研究人员希望最后能够通过测试找到一种治愈方法。

---

[1] *Histamine is a first-responder defense against invading parasites, but when turned on an allergen, it helps cause the itching, sneezing, swelling, and other nasty symptoms of allergies.
组胺是抵御外来寄生虫的第一反应者,但是如果是过敏原侵入,组胺就会协助引起过敏症的一系列烦人的症状:瘙痒、喷嚏、肿大等。

❹ A First Test of Efficacy—FAHF-1

Once the team had developed a reliable method of inducing peanut allergy in mice, it was time to test FAHF-1, the basic nine herbs of WMW with the addition of the magic mushroom *Ling Zhi* and another herb called *Zhi Fu Zi* which is "used in emergency situations in which there is a complete void of yang energy … characterized by profuse perspiration with clear and cold sweats, intolerance of cold, faint respiration, icy extremities, diarrhea containing undigested food, and faint or imperceptible pulse"[①]—in other words, shock, one of the unmistakable features of full-blown anaphylaxis.

Kamal Srivastava, PhD, who runs the animal studies, joined the team at this point. He says of the process, "At the time much of the animal work was being planned, we met with Dr. Li as a group on a weekly basis. Xiu-Min was very receptive to our suggestions and interpretation of the data, although we needed to have a good argument to convince her."

What followed was, with refinements and variations, a template for more than 10 years of experiments with mice. *[②][③] For each successive test, the mice would be sensitized using the method already described and then treated—or sham treated—in the same way so that their little bodies would respond in the same ways and provide meaningful apples-to-apples comparisons with each new test.

❹ 食物过敏中药方剂 1 号(FAHF-1)的第一次疗效测试

一旦研究人员开发了一种诱导小鼠对花生过敏的可靠方法,就是测试 FAHF-1 的时候了。WMW 包含基本的九种草药,外加上有神奇蘑菇之称的灵芝和另一种名为制附子的药物,这是"用于紧急情况下的亡阳……特征为大量出清稀冷汗,恶寒,呼吸微弱,四肢厥冷,腹泻并含有未消化食物,以及脉微欲绝"——换言之,是完全成熟的过敏反应的明确特征之一:休克。

进行动物研究的卡马尔·斯里瓦斯塔瓦博士在这个时候加入了团队。他谈到这个过程,"当时动物研究工作的大部分正在计划,我们与李秀敏博士每周碰一次面。秀敏非常接受我们对数据的建议和解释,尽管我们需要有一个好的论据来说服她。"

紧接着是为十多年小鼠研究制定的经过改进的模板。对于每个连续的测试,将使用前面描述过的方法来对小鼠进行致敏,然后再治疗或者假治疗,以相同的方式使它们的身体以相同的方式作出反应,并为每个新测试提供有意义的同类比较。

---

① http://www.aompress.com/book_herbology/pdfs/FuZi.pdf.

② *All experimental data in this chapter is drawn from the same article.
本篇中的所有实验数据都来自同一篇文章。

③ Xiu-Min L, Teng-Fei Z, Chih-Kang H, et al. Food Allergy Herbal Formula-1 (FAHF-1) blocks peanut-induced anaphylaxis in a murine model[J]. Journal of Allergy and Clinical Immunology, 2001, 108(4): 639－646.

The identical strain of five-week-old mice— "model" C3H/HeJ—was ordered as in the earlier described experiment to induce allergy along with the full menu of food and cholera toxin for inducing peanut allergy.

相同的五周龄小鼠——"模型"C3H／HeJ——按照先前描述的实验中的顺序,以诱导过敏反应的食物和霍乱毒素的全食物菜单喂食,诱导花生过敏。

Components of Herbal Medicines in FAHF-1

	TCM Materia Medica (pinyin)	Equivalent Pharmaceutical Name	Amount(g)	Part Used
1	Wu Mei	Fructus Pruni Mume	30	Fruit
2	Ling Zhi(Chi)	Ganoderma Lucidum	15	Fruiting body
3	Fu Zi(Zhi)	Radix Lateralis Aconiti Carmichaeli Praeparata	3	Root
4	Chuan Jiao	Pericarpium Zanthoxyli Bungeani	1.5	Seed
5	Xi Xin	Herba Cum Radice Asari	1	Whole
6	Huang Lian（Chuan）	Rhizoma Coptidis	9	Root
7	Huang Bai	Cortex Phellodendri	6	Root
8	Gan Jiang	Rhizoma Zingiberis	6	Root
9	Gui Zhi	Ramulus Cinnamomi Cassiae	3	Twig
10	Ren Shen（Hong）	Radix Ginseng	9	Root
11	Dang Gui(Shen)	Corpus Radix Angelica Sinensic	9	Root

FAHF-1 中的药物成分

	中药(拼音)	对应的药物名称	剂量(克)	药用部位
1	乌梅	Fructus Pruni Mume	30	果实
2	灵芝(赤灵芝)	Ganoderma Lucidum	15	子实体
3	附子(制)	Radix Lateralis Aconiti Carmichaeli Praeparata	3	根
4	川椒	Pericarpium Zanthoxyli Bungeani	1.5	籽
5	细辛	Herba Cum Radice Asari	1	全体
6	黄连(川)	Rhizoma Coptidis	9	根
7	黄柏	Cortex Phellodendri	6	根
8	干姜	Rhizoma Zingiberis	6	根
9	桂枝	Ramulus Cinnamomi Cassiae	3	枝
10	人参(红参)	Radix Ginseng	9	根
11	当归(身)	Corpus Radix Angelica Sinensic	9	根

All of the herbal medicines were ordered from the China Academy of Chinese Medical Sciences, Xiyuan Chinese Medicine Research and Pharmaceutical Manufacturer in Beijing, and inspected by pharmacists according to the Chinese Herbal Medicine Materia Medica and *Pharmacopoeia of the People's Republic of China* at the China-Japan Friendship Hospital, Beijing, China. This supplier has been used throughout the process to ensure uniformity and accountability. Each big hospital in China has its own pharmaceutical manufacturing facilities that make all the preparations used there, right down to saline solution. Although this might someday be a problem for supplying the export market for particular herbal-based drugs if demand picks up, for experimental purposes, this is not an issue; however, all medications imported undergo further quality-control testing at Mount Sinai.

FAHF-1 Preparation

This section should be read carefully by anyone who envisions do-it-yourself treatment from herbs ordered through the Internet or purchased at an apothecary in Chinatown. Imagine doing the following every day for months at a time!

The daily human adult dosage, based on figures in the *Pharmacopeia of the People's Republic of China*, was 92.5 grams (a little less than 4 ounces) of raw herbs, *decocted* (water-extracted). To begin, *Ling Zhi* and *Zhi Fu Zi* were boiled individually for 2 hours, and the decoction was filtered and lyophilized, or freeze dried, and the remaining components—*Wu Mei*, *Chuan Jiao*, *Xi Xin*, *Huang lian*, *Huang Bai*, *Gan Jiang*, *Gui Zhi*, *Ren Shen*, *Dang Gui*—were then added and boiled for an additional 1 hour. After

所有的草药都订购于北京的中国中医科学院、西苑中药研究和制药厂,并由药剂师根据《中药学》和《中华人民共和国药典》(简称《中国药典》)在北京中日友好医院进行检查。药品自始至终由该供应商提供,以确保统一性和责任性。中国每家大医院都有自己的制药设施,也做制剂,甚至包括生理盐水。尽管某天草药类药物出口市场需求增加,这可能成为供应市场的障碍,但为了实验这不是问题。然而,进口的所有药物需在西奈山进行进一步的质量控制测试。

FAHF-1 制备

所有通过互联网或唐人街的药材商来购买自己治疗用的草药的人们,应该仔细阅读这个部分。想象一下连续几个月每天都做以下事情!

根据《中国药典》的数据,成人每日的剂量为 92.5 g(略小于 4 盎司)原料药,经熬煮(水提取)后服用。开始时,将灵芝和制附子分开煎 2 小时,过滤冷冻干燥或冷冻干燥,再加入剩余成分——乌梅、川椒、细辛、黄连、黄柏、干姜、桂枝、人参、当归,再煮 1 小时。冷冻干燥并混合后,成为 15 g 约半盎司的干提取物。

lyophilizing and mixing, the yield was 15 grams of dried extract—about half an ounce. Then, using conversion table based on body surface area from another Chinese text, *Pharmacology for Experimental Studies*, a dose of 21 milligrams of freeze-dried FAHF-1 in 0.5 mL of water was administered to each mouse twice daily.

Two groups of mice were sensitized with 5 mg of peanut plus 10 micrograms of cholera toxin, administered intragastrically and boosted 1 and 3 weeks later. One week after the final sensitization dose, some of these mice were treated, receiving 21 mg of FAHF-1 or being sham-treated with water, administered by intragastric gavage twice daily for 7 weeks.

Then came the challenge for all three groups—10 mg of crude peanut extract administered intragastrically. Naïve mice served as additional controls.

Plasma was collected 30 minutes after challenge, and histamine levels were determined through use of an enzyme immunoassay kit made by a French company, which I only mention because I am intrigued by the global supply chain for science. Degranulated mast cells in ear tissues were counted in samples collected 40 minutes after the peanut challenge.

Peanut-specific serum IgE concentrations were measured along with total serum IgG and IgA. Splenocytes—cells that originate in the spleen, including T and B lymphocytes, dendritic cells and macrophages, which have different immune functions—were taken from 5 mice in each group for

然后,根据另一篇中文文章《药理实验研究》中基于人体表面积的换算表,每只小鼠喂服溶于 0.5 mL 水的 21 mg 冷冻干燥 FAHF-1,每日两次。

两组小鼠用 5mg 花生加 10μg 霍乱毒素灌胃致敏,并在 1 周和 3 周后加强。在最终致过敏剂量后一周,部分小鼠接受 21mg 的 FAHF-1 灌胃或用水进行假治疗,每天两次,共 7 周。

然后是三组都进行的测试——10mg 粗花生提取物进行灌胃。未处理组小鼠作为额外的对照。

在实验后 30 分钟收集血浆,通过使用由法国公司制造的酶免疫测定试剂盒测定组胺水平,我之所以提到这一点,是因为我对科学的全球供应链感兴趣。花生实验 40 分钟后对收集到的样本耳组织中的脱粒肥大细胞进行计数。

测定花生特异性血清 IgE 浓度以及血清总 IgG 和 IgA。从每组中选择 5 只小鼠,取其脾脏细胞,包括 T 和 B 淋巴细胞,树突状细胞和巨噬细胞,它们具有不同的免疫功能,用于培养和研究。在食物激发实验前

culture and study. Sera from treated peanut-allergic mice were obtained one day before challenge and subjected to biochemical analyses of liver- and kidney-function testing. Toxicity was measured, which was a crucial step when working with this particular set of herbs because, as was mentioned briefly earlier, a couple of the herbs did raise red flags.

Starting 30 to 40 minutes after the challenge, anaphylactic symptoms were scored.

In the sham-treated group—the ones that received the placebo—80% exhibited symptoms such as itching (score 1; 10%); puffiness around the eyes, swelling around the mouth, and diarrhea (score 2; 30%); labored respiration (score 3; 20%); and loss of consciousness or little activity after prodding (score 4; 20%). This list alone should make us grateful that mice make such effective stand-ins for people for such research. By contrast, FAHF-1-treated mice and naïve mice exhibited no symptoms after challenge.

During anaphylaxis, one of the most dangerous effects is a collapse in blood pressure, which is accompanied by lower temperatures as the heart labors to delivery blood to vital organs and extremities. This indicator should make anyone who has ever taken care of a sick child even more pleased that mice make such apt research subjects. Each mouse had its temperature taken rectally 30 minutes after the peanut challenge. Just in case you were curious about how such an undignified procedure is administered to a mouse, a 3A inch (19 mm) long probe with a ball tip 1.7 mm (0.07 inch) in diameter attached to a 5-foot cable attached to a computer.

一天收集对花生过敏小鼠的血清,并进行肝和肾功能测试的生物化学分析。测量毒性是使用这一组特定草药的关键步骤,因为如前所述,一些草药确实不符合规定。

在食物激发实验30至40分钟后开始对过敏症状进行评分。

在假治疗组中,接受安慰剂的小鼠80%表现出瘙痒的症状(评分1;10%);眼周浮肿,口腔周围肿胀和腹泻(评分2;30%);呼气困难(评分3;20%);刺激后的意识丧失或活动量少(评分4;20%)。这个列表就足以让我们应该感谢小鼠,为人类在这样的研究中做如此有效的替身。相比之下,FAHF-1治疗的小鼠和未处理的小鼠在食物激发实验后没有表现出症状。

在过敏性反应期间,最危险的影响之一是当心脏努力将血液输送到重要器官和四肢时伴随着血压降低和体温降低。这一指标应该会让任何曾经照顾过生病孩子的人更高兴,因为老鼠是如此合适的研究对象。在花生刺激30分钟后,通过直肠测量每只小鼠的体温。如果你想知道这样一个不体面的程序是如何应用到老鼠身上的,答案是一根3A英寸(19毫米)长的探针,一个直径1.7毫米(0.07英寸)的球头,连着一根5英尺长的电缆,最终连在电脑上。

By every measure, the results were encouraging. Core body temperatures showed substantial drops among the sham-treated mice, with little difference in the naïve group and the FAHF-1 treated mice.

Blood assays, too, supported the observed results.

Tissues of the sham-treated mice revealed the remains of many degranulated mast cells after the challenge, while those that had been treated showed levels not significantly above the sham group. Plasma histamine levels also were markedly elevated in the sham-treated group but not in the FAHF-1-treated group. The naïve mice had the lowest levels all.

Peanut IgE tracked these other numbers closely. When FAHF-1 treatment was initiated four weeks after sensitization, peanut-specific IgE levels were significantly higher in both sensitized groups than in the naïve group.

No more mice were sacrificed and no more treatment given, but IgE was monitored in the survivors for an additional four weeks. At the end of that time, levels were essentially the same as they had been when treatment was discontinued and were roughly half those for the sham-treated mice.

Finally, T cells from sham-treated mice produced much higher levels of the cytokines associated with allergic responses.

This was a grand slam for FAHF-1, and it was achieved with no detectable toxicity, a prerequisite for eventual approval. "First do no harm" is a part of the process.

从各个方面来看,结果都是鼓舞人心的。假治疗小鼠的核心体温显著下降,未处理组和 FAHF-1 治疗的小鼠有轻微的差异。

血液测定也支持观察到的结果。

假治疗小鼠的组织显示食物刺激后许多脱粒肥大细胞的残留物,而已经治疗的小鼠的组织显示的水平并未明显高于假治疗组。血浆组胺在假治疗组中也显著升高,但在 FAHF-1 治疗组中没有显著升高。未处理组小鼠具有最低水平。

花生 IgE 密切追踪这些其他数字。当在致敏 4 周后开始进行 FAHF-1 治疗时,两个致敏组中花生特异性 IgE 水平显著高于未处理组。

不再有小鼠死亡并且不再给予治疗,但继续监测存活小鼠 IgE 四周时间。监测结束时,IgE 水平基本上与停止治疗时的水平相同,并且大约是假治疗小鼠的一半。

最后,来自假治疗小鼠的 T 细胞产生了更高水平的与过敏反应相关的细胞因子。

这是 FAHF-1 的"大满贯",并且没有检测到毒性是最终批准的先决条件。"无损于病人为先"是整个过程的一部分。

The discussion at the end of the published article draws some interesting inferences from the results that can only excite peanut-allergy families everywhere:

In this study, we treated PN-sensitized mice with an herbal formulation and demonstrated that this treatment abrogated PN-induced anaphylactic symptoms and significantly reduced PN-specific serum IgE levels. Our results suggest that an immune system already "committed" to an anaphylactic pathway can be normalized, at least partially, after treatment with FAHF-1 in this model.

They demonstrated that the herbal formula suppressed production of Th2 cytokines, the ones associated with allergies, and speculated that it directly inhibited allergen-induced B-cell activation, "thereby reducing the number of allergen-specific molecules bound to mast cells."

Moreover—and this is very important for anyone who worries that reduced Th2, allergy-associated activity may also compromise acquired immunity to, say, polio—TH1 activity, which controls immunity to infectious disease, was unaffected.

If that is the case, that Th2 activity is reduced while Th1 is not, it means that fewer "battle-ready allergy troops" will be out there looking for a fight when the enemy—peanut proteins—present themselves with no detrimental effects for the body's ability to fight infection. The researchers also observed that the herbal formula may reduce intestinal permeability, meaning that fewer proteins will have access to the bloodstream, which is the vehicle for delivering

这篇发表的文章最后的讨论部分从结果中得出了一些有趣的推论，这些结果只会让各地的有对花生过敏的病人的家庭兴奋不已：

在这项研究中，我们用草药制剂治疗花生致敏小鼠，并表明这种治疗能消除花生诱导过敏症状和显著减少花生特异性血清 IgE 水平。我们的结果表明已经"致力于"过敏性途径的免疫系统能够在该模型中用 FAHF-1 治疗后，至少部分实现正常化。

他们证明中药方剂抑制 Th2 细胞因子（与过敏有关的细胞因子）的产生，并推测其直接抑制过敏原诱导的 B 细胞的活化作用，"从而减少与肥大细胞结合的过敏原特异性分子的数量。"

更重要的是，这对于那些担心减少 Th2 过敏相关活性也可能损害获得性免疫如脊髓灰质炎 Th1 活性的人来说是非常重要的。

如果 Th2 活性降低而 Th1 没有，这意味着当敌人花生源蛋白质本身对机体抵御感染的能力不存在有害的影响时，将有更少的"做好战斗准备的过敏部队"在那里备战。研究人员还观察到中药方剂可能降低肠道可渗透性，意味着将有更少的蛋白质进入血液，血液是将过敏原传递到多个器官系统的载体，而这些器官

allergens to the multiple organ systems whose activation defines anaphylaxis.

The paper ends on the cautious note that is frustrating to people desperate for treatment: "Although animal models are not identical to human disease and further studies regarding effects of long-term administration and/or interactions with prescription drugs are required, this study suggests that FAHF-1 might be useful for the treatment of PN allergy and perhaps of other IgE-mediated food allergies."

The results were good. Very good.

❺ Process of Elimination

For the next phase, two herbs were eliminated from FAHF-1—*Zhi Fu Zi* and *Xi Xin* (*Herba Asari*). Both are useful, like *Ling Zhi*, for treating shock.

This decision was made for several reasons. The active ingredients in these herbs are alkaloids, which means they are in a class of drugs that includes cocaine, morphine, and caffeine. This is not to imply "guilt by association," but alkaloids are tricky to use in refined forms. As you will read, refining would be imperative in the effort to turn the basic formula into manageable medication.

A better-known example of a TCM ingredient containing alkaloids that doesn't make an easy transition from its herbal state to a refined form is *Ma Huang*, which has been used by TCM practitioners to treat asthma and other conditions for thousands of years. It was highly valued in ancient China and environs, and it has been found in tombs along with other treasures.

系统的激活定义了过敏反应。

该文章结束时谨慎地提醒那些渴望得到治疗的人:"虽然动物模型与人类疾病不相同,并且需要对长期服药和/或与处方药物的相互作用进一步研究,研究结果表明 FAHF-1 可能对治疗花生过敏和其他 IgE 介导的食物过敏有效。"这一说明(让那些人)略感受挫。

结果良好,非常好。

❺ 减药过程

在下一阶段,从 FAHF-1 中除去了制附子和细辛两种草药。和灵芝一样,这两种药对治疗休克都有用。

这个决定出于几个原因。这些草药中的活性成分是生物碱,这意味着它们包括在含有可卡因、吗啡和咖啡因的一类药物中。这不是暗示"关联罪",但生物碱很难用于精炼的剂型。正如你将会看到的,精炼是努力将基本方剂变成可管理的药物的必要条件。

含有生物碱的中药成分很难从草药状态轻易转化为精炼剂型,这其中一个著名的例子就是麻黄。数千年来,麻黄一直被中医用来治疗哮喘和其他疾病。它在古代中国和周边地区受到高度重视,并在墓葬中与其他珍宝一起被发现。

The active ingredient in *Ma Huang* is ephedra, which in its synthetic version was taken orally for asthma by the early 20th century in the United States. ① (Safe asthma treatments were hard to come by in those days: "asthma cigarettes" made from the leaves of *datura stramonium*, also known as jimpson weed, a hallucinogen, were the only other remedy in common use. ②) More recently, ephedra was legally used as a diet aid (at much higher concentrations than for asthma), but it was linked to sudden death from ephedrine toxicity, nephrolithiasis, and acute hepatitis and is now banned. It is also an ingredient in the decongestant pseudoephedrine and its rogue cousin, methamphetamine.

Both Zhi Fu Zi and *Xi Xin* raised questions with the US Food and Drug Administration (FDA) because of quality-control issues, enunciated at length in a 2000 publication of Guidance for Industry for botanicals. ③ The FDA was concerned about residual aconitine ("a poisonous solid that occurs naturally in the roots and leaves of aconite plants such as monkshood and wolfsbane"④). ⑤ The scientific name of *Zhi Fu Zi* (*Radix Lateralis Aconiti Carmichaeli Praeparata*) leaves nothing to the imagination on this score.

Xi Xin was the subject of a 2001 warning on botanicals that contain aristolochic acid, which had been detected in numerous samples imported into the United States and in Europe, and was associated with

20 世纪早期,含有麻黄活性成分的合成剂在美国用于口服治疗哮喘。(安全的哮喘治疗在当时很难得:"哮喘香烟"由曼陀罗的叶子做成,也被称为吉普逊草,一种致幻剂,是唯一常用的其他疗法。)最近,麻黄被用作合法饮食辅助(浓度比治疗哮喘时高得多),但它同麻黄碱毒性、肾结石和急性肝炎猝死都有关,现在被禁用。它也是解充血药假麻黄碱及其劣种同类甲基苯丙胺的成分。

美国食品和药物管理局(FDA)提出了有关制附子和细辛质量控制的问题,这在2000年的《美国植物药产业指南》中有详细阐述。FDA关注残留乌头碱("在乌头植物的根和叶中天然存在的有毒固体,例如乌头和附子草")。制附子(*Radix Lateralis Aconiti Carmichaeli Praeparata*)的学名倒不会让人想到它有什么残留毒性。

2001 年关于含有马兜铃酸的植物药预警的主要对象是细辛,该药物在进口到美国和欧洲的许多样品中被检测到与肾衰竭有关。"当足够

---

① http://en. wikipedia. org/wiki/Ephedra.

② http://en. wikipedia. org/wiki/Datura_stramonium.

③ http://www. fda. gov/OHRMS/DOCKETS/98fr/001392gd. pdf.

④ http://www. bing. com/Dictionary/search? q = define + aconitine& qpvt = acontine&FORM = DTPDIA.

⑤ Fans of horror movies will recall that wolfsbane was used to cure people afflicted with Iycanthropy—werewolves.
恐怖电影的影迷会想起附子草(狼毒草)用来治疗变狼狂——狼人。

kidney failure. "The ingredient will only be allowed to enter the U. S. when adequate testing shows that the suspect ingredients are free of aristolochic acid."[1] *Aristolochia clematitis*, or European bloodwort, was the subject of an 2013 *New Yorker* article called "Poisoned Land." The author, Elif Batuman, says that he and his father, a kidney specialist, visited a lab that had 400 kidneys in bottles, and that his dad said he had never seen kidneys so badly shrunken. The degree of toxicity may vary according to the soil composition of particular regions where these herbs are grown.

Fortunately, based on their reading of the TCM formulation system, the team determined that neither *Zhi Fu Zi* nor *Xi Xin* was crucial to the long-term therapeutic goals of their research. If they had been, it might have been worth the time and expense of ensuring toxin-free supplies; however, the shock-protection qualities of *Zhi Fu Zi* could be achieved through "magic mushroom." *Xi Xin* primarily helped relieve stomach pain, so the researchers increased the dose of *Gan Jiang* (gingerroot) which is safe and accomplishes the same thing.

As mentioned earlier, one big challenge was to find a reliable supply of *Ling Zhi* with the requisite degree of purity for manufacture. With the help of a university professor friend, Dr. Li did manage to locate a remote, undeveloped forest where the mushroom grows wild. They compared samples from eight other regions, some of them quite close to this particular forest, and found those samples wanting.

的测试显示可疑成分不含马兜铃酸时,该成分才允许进入美国。"铁线莲状马兜铃或欧洲血藤是2013年《纽约客》杂志一篇名为《中毒的土地》的文章的主题。作者叶利夫·巴图曼说,他和他的父亲,一个肾脏病专家,参观了一个实验室,里边有若干个瓶子,共装有400个肾脏,他的父亲说,他从来没有见过这么严重萎缩的肾脏。(植物药的)毒性程度可根据这些草药生长的特定区域的土壤成分的变化而变化。

幸运的是,基于他们对中医组方体系的认识,李秀敏博士团队认为制附子或细辛对其研究的长期治疗目标都不是至关重要的。若如此,目前为止为保证无毒物料所花费的时间和金钱都是值得的。但是,制附子通过"神奇蘑菇"达到防止休克的目的。细辛主要帮助缓解胃痛,因此研究人员增加了干姜的剂量,不仅安全而且达到了同样的疗效。

如前所述,一个大的挑战就是找到具有所需纯度的灵芝的可靠供应。在大学教授朋友的帮助下,李秀敏博士设法找到一个偏远的未开发的森林,那儿有野生蘑菇。他们比较了来自其他八个地区的样,其中一些地区相当接近这个森林并在那里发现了需要的样品。

---

[1] http://www.fda.gOv/Food/DietarySupplements/Alerts/ucm096388.htm.

When food-allergy moms ask me why versions of one FAHF or another aren't widely available, seeing as how versions of them have been in use for centuries, this is the kind of thing I tell them. You can't mix these things at home out of things you find at your health-food store. Even if they were all safe, different parts of the plant are used for the different ingredients—whole fruit, seeds, roots, or twigs depending on where the active ingredients are concentrated. This is not a job for amateurs.

I also found the extent of regulatory coverage very impressive. Alternative medicine may get some slack in the gray area between supplements and medicines, but at least in this instance, government scientists are doing their job in protecting us from known adulterants. Chemists led by Dr. Nan Yang, a six-year veteran of Dr. Li's team, are responsible for, among other things, ensuring quality and purity of all medicines and extracts used in their research. The lab adheres to European standards, which are, in fact, even higher than American ones. Each new batch received from China is compared to previous ones that have been certified free of pesticides, heavy metals, and other contaminants.

The chemistry also involves isolation of active ingredients, "fingerprinting" them, studying their pharmacokinetics (what the body does to the drug, as opposed to what the drug does to the body, which is called pharmacodynamics, as defined by wikipedia), and monitoring absorption, first in cell lines, then in mice, and eventually in human subjects. Eventually, as they continue to isolate the active ingredients, they may be able to assemble these compounds in the

当食物过敏孩子的母亲问我为何 FAHF 相关配方未普及时,我告诉她们这些配方已经使用好几个世纪了。你不能把家里的这些东西与健康食品店的混淆。即使它们都是安全的,但植物的不同部位用作的成分不同——整个果实,种子,根或枝,这取决于活性成分集中的位置。这是专业性极强的工作。

我还对药品监管范围印象深刻。替代医学的补充剂和药物之间的灰色区域的监管可能会宽松一些,但至少在这种情况下,政府的科学家正在努力保护我们免受已知假冒伪劣药品的危害。在李秀敏博士团队工作了六年的杨楠博士领导的化学家们负责确保他们研究中使用的所有药物和提取物的质量和纯度。实验室实际上遵守的是甚至高于美国标准的欧洲标准。从中国收到的每个新批次药物都会与之前已经认证过的无农药、无重金属和无其他污染物的批次进行比较。

化学(实验)还包括分离活性成分,用"指纹标记"它们,研究它们的药效动力学(维基百科定义为身体对药物的作用,与药物对身体的作用相反,它被称为药物动力学),并首先监测其在细胞系中,然后在小鼠中,最终在人类受试者中的吸收。最终,当继续分离活性成分时,科学家们可能能够在实验室中聚集这些化

laboratory, but for now, we must depend on the unique combinations provided by nature.

合物,但是现在,我们必须依赖于自然生长独特的植物药组合。

❻ Proof

In 2005, Dr. Li's team published the first of two landmark studies signaling the efficacy of FAHF-2. The title of the first of these, led by Kamal D. Srivastava, who directs biological studies for the Sinai team, states the case very directly: "The Chinese Herbal Medicine Formula FAHF-2 Completely Blocks Anaphylactic Reactions in a Murine Model of Peanut Allergy."

This study included data from a series of five experiments over a period of two and a half years.[①]

The procedure was always the same. After sensitization, with boosting at 5 weeks and 7 weeks, and with sham and naïve mice as controls, all mice were challenged with ground peanut at week 10 (one week post therapy). To determine whether FAHF-2 protected against anaphylaxis for a significant period of time after therapy, mice received 6 sensitization doses at weekly intervals, followed by boosting doses at weeks 6 and 8. Mice were challenged at week 12 or 14 (3 and 5 weeks post therapy). An earlier study showed that 6 weeks after the week-8 boost was the latest time at which mice still exhibited hypersensitivity to initial challenge.

The mice were assessed for systemic anaphylaxis signs, temperature, and plasma histamine levels. In addition, immediately before the second intragastric peanut challenge, two mice from each group were

❻ 验证

2005 年,李秀敏博士的团队发表了两篇标志着 FAHF-2 疗效的里程碑式的研究文章中的第一篇。由卡马尔·D. 斯利瓦斯塔瓦指导的西奈山生物团队学研究非常直接地陈述了这个情况:"中药配方 FAHF-2 完全阻断花生过敏小鼠模型的过敏反应。"

这项研究包括的数据是从一系列的为期两年半的五个实验中获得的。

实验步骤保持不变。致敏后,在第 5 周和第 7 周加强,假治疗小鼠和未处理小鼠作为对照组,所有小鼠都在第 10 周(治疗后一周)给予花生碎。为了确定在治疗后的相当长一段时间内 FAHF-2 是否对过敏反应有保护作用,每周给予小鼠 6 次致敏剂量,随后在第 6 周和 8 第周增加剂量。小鼠在第 12 周或第 14 周(治疗后三周和五周)又用食物激发。早前的一项研究表明,第 8 周加强剂量后的六周小鼠对首次食物激发仍然表现出过敏反应。

对小鼠进行全身性过敏反应体征评估,包括体温和血浆组胺水平。此外,在第二次用花生灌胃之前,每组小鼠中有两只注射蓝染料,脚掌显

---

① Srivastava K D, Kattan J D, Sampson H A, et al. The Chinese herbal medicine formula FAHF-2 completely blocks anaphylactic reactions in a murine model of peanut allergy[J]. Journal of Allergy and Clinical Immunology, 2004, 113 (2): S337.

injected with blue dye and their footpads were examined for blue color that would indicate leakage from the capillaries—indicative of the drastically lower blood pressure that is a symptom of anaphylaxis. (Many homeowners may be familiar with this phenomenon if they rely on circulating hot water to heat their homes. In the event that the pump fails, the solder seals in the pipes may start to leak as water pressure falls. I speak from experience.)

示蓝色表明毛细血管渗漏,表示血压大幅降低,这是过敏反应的症状。(许多买房的人可能会熟悉这一现象,如果他们依靠循环热水来加热他们的家,在泵失灵的情况下,管道中的焊接密封处可能会因为水压下降开始泄漏。这是我的经验之谈。)

Incidence of Anaphylactic Reactions (across multiple experiments over 2.5 years)

	Challenge time	Sham		FAHF-2		Naïve	
		n/total	Anaphylactic score Median (Range)	n/total	Anaphylactic score (Median)	n/total	Anaphylactic score (Median)
Exp. #1	W10	9/9	3(2–4)	0/9	0***	0/9	0
Exp. #2	W12	8/8	3(2–4)	0/4	0***	0/5	0
Exp. #3	W14	8/8	3(2–3)	0/4	0**	0/5	0
Exp. #4	W14	8/8	3(2–4)	0/4	0***	0/5	0
Exp. #5	W14	5/5	3(2–3)	0/5	0***	0/5	0
Totals		38/38	3(2–4)	0/26	0###	0/29	0

过敏性反应发生率(两年半来的多次试验)

	刺激时间	假治疗组		FAHF-2 组		未经处理组	
		次数/总次数	过敏性反应得分中值(范围)	次数/总次数	过敏性反应得分(中值)	次数/总次数	过敏性反应得分(中值)
实验1	W10	9/9	3(2–4)	0/9	0***	0/9	0
实验2	W12	8/8	3(2–4)	0/4	0***	0/5	0
实验3	W14	8/8	3(2–3)	0/4	0**	0/5	0
实验4	W14	8/8	3(2–4)	0/4	0***	0/5	0
实验5	W14	5/5	3(2–3)	0/5	0***	0/5	0
总计		38/38	3(2–4)	0/26	0###	0/29	0

Body Temperatures
体温

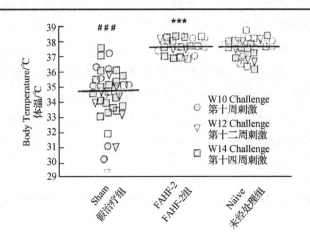

Plasma Histamine
血浆组胺

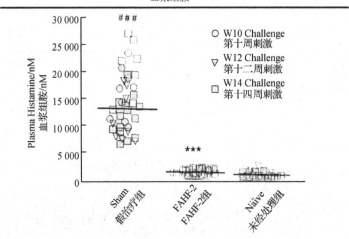

Regulation of Cytokines by Splenocytes
脾细胞的细胞因子调节

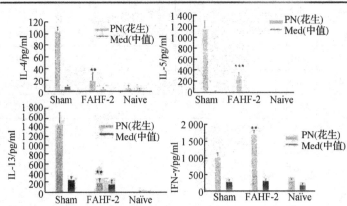

The results were dramatic. After challenge at week 10 (1 week post therapy), all sham-treated mice developed anaphylactic reactions, with a median score of 3. In contrast, FAHF-2-treated mice exhibited no anaphylactic signs. The same results were found after week-12 and -14 challenges.

Dr. Sampson asked that the experiment should be repeated, and it was done five times, all told, over a two-and-a-half-year period. The pooled data show that all 38 sham-treated mice developed anaphylaxis, with a median anaphylactic score of 3, indicating a severe anaphylactic reaction. In contrast, none of the 26 FAHF-2-treated mice and none of 29 naïve mice developed anaphylaxis after challenge. These results demonstrated that FAHF-2 "has potent protective properties" against peanut-induced anaphylaxis and that the complete protection was consistent and relatively persistent. Plasma histamine and IgE levels were all consistent with efficacy of FAHF-2.

Just as dramatic were the figures for loss of body temperature. Mouse normal, just above 37 degrees Celsius, is essentially the same as human normal. For all the challenges in all experiments, the median loss of temperature was more than two degrees Celsius (to 95 degrees Fahrenheit) for the sham-treated mice, which is essentially the lower limit for normal metabolism and bodily function. ① Those for the treated and naïve groups were normal.

Meanwhile, the feet of the sham-treated mice showed a distinct blue tint from capillary leakage,

结果是戏剧性的。在第 10 周（治疗后一周）测试之后，所有假治疗的小鼠发生过敏反应，中值评分为 3。相比之下，FAHF-2 治疗的小鼠没有表现出过敏症状。在第 12 周和第 14 周后发现相同的结果。

桑普森博士要求重复实验，并且在两年半的时间里进行了五次。汇总的数据显示，所有 38 只假治疗的小鼠发生过敏反应，中值过敏评分为 3，显示为严重过敏反应。相比之下，26 只经过 FAHF-2 处理的小鼠和 29 只未处理小鼠中没有一只在测试后发生过敏反应。这些结果证明 FAHF-2 针对花生诱导的过敏有较强的保护作用，并且完全保护作用具有一致性和相对持久性。血浆组胺和 IgE 水平都与 FAHF-2 的功效一致。

体温下降的数据变化很大。小鼠的体温正常是刚刚高于 37 摄氏度，基本上与人类正常体温相同。对于所有实验中的食物激发测试，假治疗小鼠的体温中值下降超过 2 摄氏度（至 95 华氏度），这基本上是正常代谢和身体功能的下限。治疗组和未处理组的体温正常。

同时，假治疗小鼠的脚掌显示毛细血管渗漏明显的蓝色，而经 FAHF-

① http://en. wikipedia. org/wiki/Normal_human_body_temperature.

while the FAHF-2 mice were indistinguishable from the naïve.

In 2007, Dr. Li and a team of four other researchers published the second of these watershed critical studies, titled "Induction of Tolerance after Establishment of Peanut Allergy by the Food Allergy Herbal Formula-2 Is Associated with Up-Regulation of Interferon-γ."[①] Interferon-gamma (IFN-γ) is a cytokine with known anti-allergenic properties, secreted by the Th1 helper cells. Up-Regulation is a good thing for reducing the severity of the allergic response; the greater the output of the Th1 cells compared to Th2, the less allergic the patient will be.

The article also provides another glimpse of the continually fascinating—to me, anyway—commercial supply chain that supports laboratory research. This work can't be done with materials from your local pet shop, pharmacy, and hardware stores. All procedures and the paraphernalia required to perform them are documented in the peer-reviewed article. If the proof of an experiment is that it must be replicable, following this template, you should be able to do the same thing at home, if you have the requisite thousands of dollars of equipment and skills.

Once again, an order went out to Jackson Labs.

The rest of the inventory included freshly ground whole roasted peanut and crude peanut extract (CPE),

2 处理过的小鼠与未处理组无区别。

2007 年,李秀敏博士和另外四位研究人员发表了第二篇标志着领域转折点的文章,名为《食物过敏中药方剂 2 确立的花生过敏后诱发耐受性与干扰素上调有关》。干扰素-γ(IFN-γ)是具有已知的抗过敏性能的细胞因子,由 Th1 辅助细胞分泌。上调是减少过敏反应;Th1 细胞与 Th2 相比的输出越大,患者的过敏反应越少。

这篇文章还提供了另一种视角,让我们得以一窥支持实验室研究的商业供应链——无论如何,对我来说是很有吸引力的。研究对象不能从当地宠物店、药店和五金店引进。研究所需的所有程序和工具都记录在同行评审的文章中。如果实验证明它一定是可复制的,你应该能根据这个方法在家里做同样的事情,只要你有数千美元的设备和技能。

(研究小组)又向杰克逊实验室下了订单。

其余的存货包括新鲜烤花生和花生粗提取物(CPE),霍乱毒素,也

---

① Qu C, Srivastava K, Ko J, et al. Induction of tolerance after establishment of peanut allergy by the food allergy herbal formula-2 is associated with up-regulation of interferon-γ[J]. Clinical and Experimental Allergy, 2007, 37(6): 846 – 855.

cholera toxin. There were also numerous pieces of specialized apparatus.

An ample supply of FAHF-2 formula was secured from a certified medical herb facility in Beijing and its quality controlled according to the standards of Pharmacopoeia of China.

Blood samples were obtained from tail veins before sensitization began and throughout the process. Sera were collected and stored at −80 degrees Celsius (−176 degrees Fahrenheit) until analyzed to determine levels of peanut-specific IgE, which indicates sensitization to allergens. These would provide snapshots of changes in immune activity along the way.

As before, after a peanut-free diet for the first 5 weeks of their lives, some of the mice were initiated into a crash course of life-threatening allergies while a control group of mice were left naïve (not given peanuts at all). For the peanut group, normal food was supplemented with 10 mg of ground peanuts weekly for 5 weeks, with subsequent boosting at the rate of 50 mg—all delivered directly into the stomach via a feeding tube.

After completing the week-8 boosting protocol, 8 mice—4 naïve and 4 peanut-sensitized—were given an extra-large dose of peanut (200 mg) and then observed.

After 30 minutes, 3 of the sensitized mice had 2 symptoms, and the 4th had 3 symptoms, while the naïve mice had none. All 4 allergic mice had subnormal body temperature, while the nonallergic ones were all normal. The blood showed, sure

有许多专门的设备。

FAHF-2 配方的充足供应来自一家在北京注册的中草药工厂,其质量按照《中国药典》的标准进行控制。

在致敏开始前到整个过程中,从小鼠尾静脉获得血液样本。收集血清,保存在零下80摄氏度(零下176华氏度)直到确定了花生特异性IgE水平,以此表明过敏原的致敏作用。这将提供实验过程中免疫活性变化的参照。

像以前一样,在小鼠生命中的第一个五周无花生饮食后,一些小鼠开始进入一个致命的过敏过程,而一个对照组的小鼠是未处理的(没有喂食花生)。对于花生组小鼠,在正常饮食基础上,每周补充10毫克花生碎,持续五周,随后提高到50毫克,全部直接通过饲管输入胃。

完成第8周的增加剂量后,8只小鼠中的4只未处理的和4只花生致敏的都被喂食超大剂量花生(200毫克),然后进行观察。

30分钟后,致敏组小鼠中的3只有两种症状,第4只有三种症状,而未处理组的小鼠没有症状。过敏小鼠的体温低于正常值,而非过敏小鼠体温都是正常的。果然,血液显示

enough, plasma histamine levels at combat strength in the highly allergic mice. Serum peanut-specific IgE levels—the antibodies primed for the appearance of peanut proteins—had also been high. This indicated that T-cell activity had created an imbalance between Th1 and Th2. Greater Th2 output had skewed the immune system toward allergic activity.

Clearly, the sensitized mice had been highly allergic and the naïve mice had not.

Time to Commence Treatment

FAHF-2 was administered intragastrically twice daily for 7 weeks. An additional group of peanut-allergic mice received only an equal amount of water (sham treatment). Finally, the naïve mice served as controls. All mice received peanut challenges (200 mg/mouse) 24 hours after the completion of therapy at week 14 and again 4 weeks later. Cholera toxin as a mucosal adjuvant was coadministered with peanut at all times except during the final challenge. Anaphylactic-reaction scores and body temperatures were determined approximately 30 minutes following each challenge. Immediately following the final peanut challenge and evaluation of reactions, mice were killed and lymphocytes from the spleen and lymph nodes were isolated for study. [1]

高度过敏小鼠的血浆组胺水平非常高。血清花生特异性 IgE 水平——为花生蛋白质的出现做好准备的抗体——也高。这表明，T 细胞的活性造成了 Th1 和 Th2 的失衡。更大的 Th2 输出使得小鼠的免疫系统更具有过敏活性。

显然，致敏小鼠已经高度过敏，而未处理组的小鼠没有。

开始治疗

用 FAHF-2 灌胃，每天两次，持续七周。额外一组花生过敏小鼠只接受等量的水（假治疗）。最后，未处理组的小鼠作为对照组。所有的小鼠在第 14 周和第 18 周完成治疗 24 小时后，接受花生刺激（每只小鼠 200 毫克）。除了最后一次刺激，霍乱毒素作为佐剂连同花生同时喂食小鼠。每次刺激约 30 分钟后，进行过敏反应评分并测量体温。随即进行最终的花生刺激和反应评价，然后杀死小鼠，对脾脏和淋巴结的淋巴细胞进行分离研究。

---

[1] Following the final challenge, splenocytes and mesenteric lymph node (MLN) cells derived from each group were isolated by gently grinding spleens or MLNs using a syringe plunger and were strained through nylon (BD Biosciences, Bedford, MA, USA). After lysis— deconstruction—of red blood cells, splenocytes or MLN cells were resuspended in RPMI 1640 "series of media using a bicarbonate buffering system and alterations in the amounts of amino acids and vitamins" supplemented with 10% FBS (fetal bovine serum). Cells were cultured, and after 72 hours, liquids also known as supernatants were separated from the various cytokines, including IL-4, IL-5, IL- 13, IL-10, TGF-β, and IFN-γ. These were measured using the ELISA test determined by ELISA in triplicate according to the manufacturer's instructions using companies in three different states for particular components (R&D Systems, Minneapolis, MN, USA, for IL-13; Promega, Madison, WI, USA, for TGF-b; and BD Pharmin- gen, San Diego, CA, USA, for all others).

Although these cells can survive for a time outside the host, the numbers that circulate in the blood are not sufficient for test-tube research, so, using a method employed by British researchers,[①] the team cloned the lymphocytes collected from the blood of each group until they had a workable concentration. The team then separated the lymphocytes into *aliquots*—identical small portions—allowing for precise comparison of uniform samples.

These were cultured with peanut antigen to show which ones would produce Th1-IFN-γ cytokines indicating immunity or Th2 interleukins indicating allergy.

Finally, all the observed results and numbers were analyzed according to various standard methods.

The data were unambiguous. Peanut-hypersensitive mice that received FAHF-2 treatment were completely protected against anaphylactic reactions following the challenge, and their body temperatures were in the normal range, whereas all sham-treated mice exhibited anaphylactic reactions and had core body temperatures significantly lower than those of naïve mice. And, unlike as in corticosteroid therapy, there was no evidence of reduced immunity to infections. As Dr. Engler points out: "This is what is so profoundly new about this therapy—a steroid-like action against allergic inflammation without compromising infection defense *and* persistence of the effect, in contrast to steroid, where tapering is associated with the problem flaring again."

虽然这些细胞可以在宿主体外存活一段时间,但循行在血液的细胞数量不足以进行试管研究。因此,采用英国研究者的方法,研究小组克隆从各组小鼠血液中收集的淋巴细胞,直到有一个可行的细胞浓度。该团队将淋巴细胞等分为相同的小部分,用于统一样本的精确比较。

这些细胞是与花生抗原一起培养的,显示哪些会产生提示免疫性的 Th1-IFN-γ 细胞因子,哪些会产生指示过敏的 Th2 白介素。

最后,根据各种标准方法对所观察到的结果和数字进行了分析。

数据是明确的。花生过敏小鼠获得 FAHF-2 治疗后能完全防止花生刺激后的过敏反应,它们的体温在正常范围内,而所有的假治疗小鼠表现出过敏反应和核心体温明显低于正常小鼠。而且,没有证据表明像皮质类固醇激素治疗那样降低对感染的免疫力。恩格勒博士指出:"这种治疗方法非常新颖,像用类固醇治疗过敏一样,无须因为疗效持久而牺牲抗感染的能力,但和类固醇疗法相异的是,随着药量减少,病症不会复发。"

① Victor T, Soheila J M, Gideon L. Characterization of lymphocyte responses to peanuts in normal children, peanut-allergic children, and allergic children who acquired tolerance to peanuts[J]. Journal of Clinical Investigation, 2003, 111(7): 1065－1072.

All sham-treated mice continued to develop anaphylactic reactions following the second post-therapy challenge at week 18, whereas no anaphylactic reactions were observed in those treated with FAHF-2-treated mice. These results demonstrated that FAHF-2-established tolerance persisted for at least 4 weeks after therapy.

The observed results were borne out by the laboratory findings. FAHF-2 treatment suppressed histamine release in peanut-allergic mice. Plasma histamine levels were markedly elevated in all peanut-sensitized, sham-treated mice at week 14 following peanut challenge, while treated sensitized mice had significantly lower histamine levels effectively indistinguishable from those of naïve mice following both post-therapy challenges.

FAHF-2 also reduced peanut-specific IgE levels and increased peanut-specific IgG2a levels in peanut-allergic mice. Again, like IgG4 in humans, IgG2a is a "blocking antibody" that prevents allergens from triggering an allergic reaction. These antibodies compete with IgE for receptor space on effector cells, either mast cells or basophils. As Th2 activity diminishes, a higher proportion of IgG antibodies occupy the available mast cell openings. With a half-life of just two days, the disenfranchised IgE antibodies circulating in the blood have a brief shot at finding a perch.

The short half-life of serum IgE is important because it accounts for the unreliability of blood IgE tests. Children with no history of allergy can show high allergen-specific IgE levels as measured by a

所有的假治疗组小鼠在第 18 周接受第二次治疗后刺激，之后仍有过敏反应，而 FAFH-2 治疗的小鼠没有观察到过敏反应。这些结果表明，FAHF-2 建立的耐受性至少可持续到治疗后四周。

所得观察结果均可由实验检查证实。FAHF-2 治疗花生过敏小鼠能抑制组胺释放。花生刺激后第 14 周，所有接受花生致敏、假治疗小鼠的血浆组胺水平显著升高，而经过治疗的致敏小鼠组胺水平显著较低，与经食物刺激的未处理小鼠相比，血浆组胺水平无明显区别。

FAHF-2 也降低了花生特异性 IgE 水平，增加花生过敏小鼠 IgG2a 的水平。还是和人类的 IgG4 一样，IgG2a 是一个"封闭抗体"，能阻止过敏原引发过敏反应。这些抗体与效应细胞、肥大细胞或嗜碱性粒细胞上的 IgE 受体进行空间竞争。当 Th2 活性减弱，较高比例的 IgG 抗体占据可用肥大细胞。因为半衰期只有两天，IgE 抗体在短暂的时间内要在血液循环中找到一个栖息地。

血清 IgE 的半衰期很重要，因为它可以验证血清 IgE 测验是否可靠。无过敏史的儿童进行放射过敏原吸附试验（RAST）也会出现过敏原相

radioallergosorbent test [RAST], sending their parents into a panic. The circulating IgE antibodies can't do any damage unless they have attached themselves to effector cells, however. Once the antibodies find a place to hang their hats (i. e., on a mast cell or a basophil) they have a half-life of 6 to 8 weeks, which makes them a threat for triggering a reaction when the right allergen comes along. SPTs are more reliable than RAST because the IgE is situated on the mast cells in the skin and will prompt a local reaction.[①] SPTs are relatively safe because the skin is isolated from the blood stream, so a skin reaction will only rarely spread from the skin and involve other organ systems in an anaphylactic reaction. Anaphylaxis is generally defined as an allergic reaction in two or more organ systems, such as the skin, the digestive tract, and, most dangerously, the airways.

Before treatment (week 8), all peanut-sensitized mice had similar peanut-specific IgE levels. After treatment, however, these levels were significantly reduced. At the time of first post-challenge (week 14) measurement, treated mice showed much lower IgE than did the sham-treated mice, and the level remained significantly lower 4 weeks later (week 18). In fact, the reduction appeared more pronounced at week 18 than at week 14, demonstrating persistent suppression of IgE production. Keep in mind that the life expectancy of a lab mouse is two years. If the same level of protection holds true for humans, each 4-week period would amount to about 3 years.

IgG2a levels were significantly higher in FAHF-2-

关性高 IgE 水平,这使他们的父母陷入恐慌中。循环 IgE 抗体不能造成任何损害,除非它们依附于效应细胞。一旦抗体找到了可以依靠的地方(即在肥大细胞或嗜碱性粒细胞上),它们有一个 6 至 8 周的半衰期,这使得它们成为合适的过敏原出现时触发反应的威胁。皮肤点刺试验比放射过敏原吸附试验更可靠,因为 IgE 附着于皮肤肥大细胞,会促使产生局部反应。皮肤点刺试验是相对安全的,因为皮肤与血液分离,所以很少从皮肤和参与过敏反应的其他器官系统传播。过敏反应一般是指在两个或多个器官系统的过敏反应,如在皮肤上、消化道中,而最危险的,是在气管。

在治疗前(第 8 周),所有花生致敏小鼠有相似花生特异性 IgE 水平。然而治疗后,这些含量显著降低。第一次花生刺激后(第 14 周)测量,治疗的小鼠比假治疗的小鼠表现出较低的 IgE,其含量明显低于四周后(第 18 周)。事实上,第 18 周的减少似乎比第 14 周更明显,表明 IgE 的产生持续被抑制。要知道实验室小鼠的寿命是两年。如果人们能维持相同保护水平的话,每四周的时间都等于三年左右。

两周的 FAHF-2 治疗后(第 10

---

① Ehrlich, et al., op cit., p. 114.

treated allergic mice compared with sham-treated allergic mice following 2 weeks of FAHF-2 treatment (week 10) and remained significantly higher up to 4 weeks after therapy was complete (week 18), indicating that FAHF-2 also had a persistent effect on IgG2a production.

The Effect on T-helper Cells

The next step was to measure the effect of FAHF-2 on cytokine profiles. Clearly, FAHF-2 seemed to be effective, but why? What effects on the various proteins appear to be involved in establishing efficacy? It's a bit like taking a census; an urban planner may note changes in the life of a city— changing crime rates in different neighborhoods, school enrollments rising and falling, fire alarms, both real and false—but there's nothing like a census to understand what lies behind the changes. Likewise, it's not enough to show that a treatment like FAHF-2 works. You have to know why. What are the specific mechanisms by which it heals? What clues lie in the cell counts that might point to further improvements in the formula, and also what complications?

In a healthy immune system, there is equilibrium between Th1 activity and Th2. As I explained earlier, with allergies, there is disproportionate Th2 output, resulting in excessive IgE—ten times or more normal levels in a very allergic person. With autoimmune disorders, the imbalance tips the other way. The body essentially loses tolerance to some of its own tissues and attacks them as if they were foreign. [①]

周），经 FAHF-2 治疗的过敏小鼠 IgG2a 水平明显高于假治疗的过敏小鼠，并且这种增高持续到治疗后的四周（第 18 周），表明 FAHF-2 对 IgG2a 的产生有长效作用。

对辅助性 T 细胞的影响

下一步是测量 FAHF-2 对细胞因子的影响。显然，FAHF-2 似乎是有效的，为什么呢？对各种蛋白质的影响似乎能参与建立疗效？这有点像人口普查；城市规划师可能会注意到在一个城市生活的变化——不同社区的犯罪率的变化，学校入学率的上升和下降，火灾警报的真假，但没有什么能像普查一样了解变化背后的原因。同样，仅仅证明 FAHF-2 治疗的有效性是不够的。你必须知道原因。它治愈的具体机制是什么？细胞计数中有哪些线索可能表明方剂的进一步改善，有没有什么并发症？

在健康的免疫系统中，Th1 活性和 Th2 之间保持平衡。就像我之前解释的，过敏后，有不成比例的 Th2 输出，导致过敏者体内产生过多的 IgE，严重过敏者体内存在十倍或更多的含量。出现自体免疫失调后，人体不平衡会以另一种方式呈现。人体对自身的一些组织基本上会失去耐受性，且这些组织会像异物一样被人体攻击。

---

① Bellanti J A, et al. Immunology IV: clinical applications in health and disease [M]. Washington, DC: I Care Press, 2012.

The same disproportion of Th2 activity pertains with all allergies, not just food. That is why research on the body chemistry of allergic rhinitis and asthma can help explain the action of FAHF-2 on food allergies as well.

In a 2009 article on her work with asthma treatment, Dr. Li and her coauthor wrote:

Th1 and Th2 responses are felt to be mutually antagonistic, such that they normally exist in equilibrium and cross-regulate each other. An optimum Th1-Th2 balance has been suggested as necessary to maintain healthy immune homeostasis. Loss of such balance has been hypothesized to underlie allergic asthma through a shift in immune responses from a Th1 (IFN-γ) pattern toward a Th2 (IL-4, IL-5, and IL-13) profile, which promotes IgE production; eosinophilic inflammation, activation, and survival; and enhanced airway smooth muscle contractility. [1]

One established method of determining the prevalence of Th1 and Th2 activity is to harvest and culture cells from organs where large numbers of these lymphocytes are created. The spleen, which produces *splenocytes*, and the *mesenteric lymph nodes*, which produce MLN cells, are rich sources for gathering these cells. An abundance of the cytokines IL-4, IL-5, and IL-13, all interleukins, would show more activity by Th2 cells associated with allergies. More interferon gamma, or IFN-γ, and TGF-β (transforming growth factor beta, which controls proliferation, cellular

Th2 活性同样涉及其他过敏原，不只是食物。这就是为什么对过敏性鼻炎和哮喘的人体化学研究可以帮助解释 FAHF-2 治疗食物过敏的作用。

在 2009 年一篇关于治疗哮喘的文章中，李秀敏博士和她的合著者这样写道：

Th1 和 Th2 反应被认为是相互对立的，这样，它们通常彼此平衡和相互调节。最佳 Th1-Th2 平衡是维持健康免疫内环境稳态的必要条件之一。假设 Th1-Th2 失衡，则可通过将免疫反应从 Th1（IFN-γ）型转移至 Th2（IL-4、IL-5、IL-13）型而引起过敏性哮喘，从而促进 IgE 的产生，嗜酸性粒细胞的炎症、激活和生存，并增强气道平滑肌收缩性。

有一个已确立的方法用来确定 Th1 和 Th2 活性的患病率，那就是从产生大量淋巴细胞的器官中收集和培养细胞。产生脾细胞的脾脏和产生 MLN 细胞的肠系膜淋巴结是聚集这些细胞的丰富来源。大量的细胞因子 IL-4、IL-5、IL-13 和所有的白细胞介素将显示更多的与过敏有关的 Th2 细胞活性。γ-干扰素，或 IFN-γ 和 TGF-β 越多（转化生长因子 β，

---

[1] Li, Brown, op cit. p. 301.

differentiation, and other functions in most cells, as well as IL-10 levels) would indicate greater Th1 activity.

As predicted, MLN cells and splenocytes from FAHF-2-treated mice produced significantly less IL-4, IL-5, and IL-13 than their counterparts from sham-treated mice. MLN cells and splenocytes from FAHF-2-treated mice produced significantly greater amounts of IFN-γ.

No differences in TGF-β production were detected in FAHF-2-treated mice when compared with the sham-treated group, whereas small but significant decreases were observed in IL-10 levels. The most pronounced effect of FAHF-2 on Th1 and Th2 responses was on MLN cells in which IFN-γ production was increased up to tenfold. This finding was consistent in two separate experiments.

At this point, I must tell readers that if they are frustrated by the continual addition of new terminology, particularly that created by the accretion of letters, some in Greek and some in English, and numbers, I share your discontents. These appear from nowhere in successive published articles as we get deeper into the biochemistry. In conversations with MDs, I found that when these individuals are not specially trained in immunology, there's no special reason for them to know what I am talking about either.

Interpreting the Data

At this stage in an experiment, the researchers sit down and analyze what has been proven, what has not, and what remains to be done. In this study, they "found that FAHF-2 treatment initiated when

控制大多数细胞的细胞增殖、细胞分化和其他功能,以及 IL-10 水平)表明 Th1 活性越高。

据预测,用 FAHF-2 治疗过的小鼠 MLN 细胞和脾细胞中产生的 IL-4、IL-5 和 IL-13 明显低于假治疗的小鼠。用 FAHF-2 治疗过的小鼠的 MLN 细胞和脾细胞产生更多的 IFN-γ。

经检测,经 FAHF-2 治疗过的小鼠与假治疗组相比,在 TGF-β 产生上无差异,但 IL-10 含量显著降低。对 Th1 和 Th2 反应最明显的影响是,在 MLN 细胞中 IFN-γ 的产生增加至 10 倍。在两个独立的实验中,这一发现是一致的。

在这一点上,我必须告诉读者,如果他们受到不断增加的新术语的困扰,特别是通过字母的堆积而产生的,有希腊语、英语和数字,我和你们一样有同样的不满。随着我们对生物化学研究的深入,这些在连续发表的文章中无处不在。在与医学博士们的交谈中,我发现当这些人没有受过专门的免疫学培训时,他们也不知道我在说什么。

数据解释

在这个实验阶段,研究人员坐下来分析什么是已经证实的,什么还没有证实,什么要去证实。在这项研究中,他们发现"FAHF-2 治疗在过敏

hypersensitivity was fully established completely protected peanut-allergic mice from anaphylaxis, and that this protection persisted for at least 4 weeks after discontinuing therapy. " The " results indicated that FAHF-2 *may* prove to be of therapeutic value for peanut-allergic patients" (emphasis added). More studies would explore how long this protective effect persists.

On key measures, FAHF-2 treatment was shown to have completely blocked histamine release, which was consistent with FAHF-2's prevention of anaphylactic reactions. The researchers found that peanut-specific IgE levels began to decline about 2 weeks after treatment began and were significantly reduced immediately after completing treatment (week 14). These levels remained significantly depressed 4 weeks after therapy ceased(week 18) as compared with sham treatment, suggesting that suppressed peanut-specific IgE production may be associated with protection against peanut anaphylaxis. Interestingly, although FAHF-2 treatment did not eliminate peanut-specific IgE, it still produced complete clinical protection against anaphylaxis and completely blocked histamine release. " Therefore, the protective effect of FAHF-2 in peanut-induced anaphylaxis cannot be explained solely by the reduction of peanut-specific IgE. "

Several mechanisms appear to play additional roles in the FAHF-2 protective effect. Levels of IgG2a were increased significantly beginning 2 weeks after treatment was initiated. That was before peanut-specific IgE began to fall, and the IgG2a levels remained significantly elevated up to 4 weeks post therapy. "Thus, the enhancement of peanut-specific IgG2a levels

完全建立时开始,完全保护花生过敏小鼠不受过敏反应的影响,而这保护在停止治疗后持续至少 4 周。""结果表明,FAHF-2 可能对花生过敏患者具有治疗价值"(强调)。更多的研究将探索这种保护作用能持续多久。

在关键测量标准上,FAHF-2 治疗显示能够完全阻止组胺释放,这符合 FAHF-2 对过敏反应的预防。研究人员发现,开始治疗约两周后,花生特异性 IgE 水平开始下降,并且在完成治疗(第 14 周)后显著降低。同假治疗组相比,在治疗停止后四周(第 18 周)仍保持着对这些水平的抑制,类似于安慰剂效应,这表明抑制的花生免疫球蛋白产生物可能与防止花生过敏反应有关。有趣的是,尽管 FAHF-2 治疗并未消除花生免疫球蛋白产生物,但它仍然产生完整的临床保护来抗过敏反应并完全阻止组胺释放。"因此,FAHF-2 对于花生诱发过敏反应的保护作用,无法仅仅解释为花生免疫球蛋白的减少。"

好几种机制在 FAHF-2 保护作用中扮演额外的角色。开始治疗两周后 IgG2a 水平显著增加。花生免疫球蛋白开始下降之前,在治疗四周后 IgG2a 水平仍然显著升高。"因此,花生 IgG2a 水平的提高也可能与保护花生过敏小鼠免受过敏反应有

also may be involved in protecting peanut-allergic mice from anaphylactic reactions." FAHF-2 protection may also be associated with its effect on other effector cells such as mast cells and basophils. This possibility suggested further experiments.

There's something both exhilarating and annoying about studies like this one. The exhilaration stems from the promising results. For something as mysterious as a life-threatening allergy to " America's food "—the peanut and all its derivatives—the prospect of a cure is tantalizing. Moreover, the idea that the counter-magic can be proven not only in the achievement of tolerance but also by counting cells and assaying biochemistry leads us to hope. But evidence does not make for unequivocal assertions of victory. The results are only promising. The mouse results must be hedged—this *may* work. More work lies ahead.

❼ Whole Greater Than the Sum of Its Parts

When a compound containing many ingredients is shown to be effective, science demands that its parts be tested to show whether one or more can achieve a comparable result. Each ingredient you can drop from the final product reduces complexity and the expense of eventual manufacture. The Mount Sinai team did a study published in 2008[①] to test each herb using the same strain of mice, sensitization, and challenge protocols as the complete FAHF-2. However, the presence of an individual component may be crucial not for what it does in and of itself, but by increasing the bioavailability (effective absorption) of another—that is, the effective

关。"FAHF-2 的保护效果也可能与其他效应细胞有关,例如肥大细胞和嗜碱性粒细胞等。这种可能性有待进一步的实验(证实)。

像这样的研究既令人振奋又令人烦恼。兴奋来源于有希望的结果。对神秘的危及生命的且具有过敏性的"美国食品"——花生及其种种制成品——治愈的前景是非常诱人的。另外,"反制魔法"不仅可以在实现耐受性方面得到证明,而且还可以通过计数细胞和分析生物化学来证明,这一想法将我们引向了希望。但是证据并不能证明胜利是明确的,结果只是有希望的。小鼠实验结果肯定是两面性的——即可能是有效的。还有更多的工作要做。

❼ 整体大于部分之和

当含有多种成分的某种化合物被证明有效时,科学要求测定其中一种或多种成分是否能够达到类似的效果。因为从最终产品中每去掉一种成分都减少了最终制造的复杂性和成本。2008 年,西奈山医院研究小组公布了一项研究,该研究采用相同品系的小鼠、同样的致敏和刺激方案测定每种草药和完整的 FAHF-2。然而,单个成分自身的作用可能并不是关键的,但是它能够提高另一种成分的生物利用度(有效吸收)——即,活性化合物的有

① Jacob D K, Kamal D S, Zhong M Z, et al. Pharmacological and immunological effects of individual herbs in the Food Allergy Herbal Formula-2 (FAHF-2) on peanut allergy[J]. Phytotherapy Research, 2008, 22(5): 651-659.

absorption of an active compound—or individual components may influence different pathways individually but unlock a productive response only together.

Phellodendron chinense achieved the best results with three of four mice; however, no individual herb treatment reproduced the broad-based immunological effects of FAHF-2, including suppression of IgE and the Th2 cytokines that signal its production, and elevation of the Th1, which produces the beneficial IFN-γ and antibody IgG2a. Some individual herbs appeared to suppress peanut-stimulated-Th2 cytokine production in splenocytes.

For example, *Phellodendron chinense* treatment appeared to suppress Th2 cytokines IL-4 and perhaps IL-13, but not IL-5, whereas *Angelica Sinensis* and *Panax Ginseng* treatment appeared to decrease two of the three. *Phellodendron chinense*, although the most effective single herb overall, was insufficient as a stand-alone treatment. In later experiments, *Phellodendrm chinense* lost its effectiveness over repeated peanut challenges, in contrast to FAHF-2, which protected against anaphylaxis in several challenges over 6 months.

效吸收——或者单个成分可能分别影响各个路径,而只有合在一起才会表现出一种富有成效的反应。

黄柏在 3/4 的小鼠中达到了最好的实验结果;然而,单一草药治疗并没有产生 FAHF-2 的广泛免疫学效果,其中包括抑制 IgE 和标志其产生的 Th2 细胞因子水平以及提高产生有益 IFN-γ 和抗体 IgG2a 的 Th1 水平。不过,一些单一草药似乎可以抑制脾脏细胞中受花生刺激产生的 Th2 细胞因子。

例如,黄柏治疗表现出对 Th2 细胞因子 IL-4 的抑制作用,对 IL-13 的可能抑制作用,但对 IL-5 没有抑制作用,而当归和人参则表现出对其中两种有降低作用。尽管黄柏是最有效的单一草药,但是它不足以用作单一治疗。随后的实验中,黄柏在重复的花生刺激下丧失了有效性,而 FAHF-2 在长达 6 个月的几种刺激下始终有效。

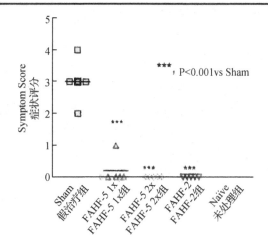

Blocking Anaphylaxis:1ˢᵗ challenge
阻断过敏性反应: 第一次刺激

Because no single herb was effective, a simplified food allergy herbal formula (sFAHF), which included *Phellodendri Chinensis*, *Zingiber officinalis*, and *Ganoderma Lucidum*, was also investigated. These three herbs collectively showed the most favorable responses in protection from anaphylaxis, suppression of IgE, and modulation of Th2/Th1 cytokines, presenting a potentially simpler alternative to FAHF-2; however, sFAHF prevented anaphylactic symptoms in only 3 of 5 mice, and plasma histamine levels were not significantly reduced after challenge.

After analyzing all 10 herbs in this way, the authors concluded, "Taken together the results suggest that all the herbs of FAHF-2 are likely required for the ability to provide complete and lasting protection against anaphylaxis and alter Th2/Th1 immune responses in a manner beneficial for therapy of food allergy."

More on the Magic in the "Magic Mushroom"

This science is not necessarily sequential. Although clinical investigations proceed in a careful stepwise manner to avoid unnecessary harm to patients, other aspects of the science, particularly delving into the mechanisms behind the effects, can be investigated by whoever has a hypothesis worth testing and the funds to do it. Dr. Li's group knew that some substances in the mushroom *Ling Zhi* are potentially bioactive (such as the steroid-related substances called triterpenes), but which ones were important in the mushroom's anti-allergy properties? They explored this question in a paper (unpublished as of this writing) with the evocative title "Ganoderic Acid C1 Isolated from *Ganoderma Lucidum* Suppresses Macrophage and

因为单一草药没有效果，所以一种简化的食物过敏中药方剂（sFAHF）应运而生，该配方包含黄柏、干姜和灵芝。在预防过敏反应、抑制 IgE 水平和调节 Th2/Th1 细胞因子方面，这三种草药均表现出良好的效果，是一种潜在的可以替代 FAHF-2 的更简单的选择；但是，sFAHF 仅能使 3/5 的小鼠不产生过敏反应，并且小鼠接受刺激后，血浆组胺水平并没有显著降低。

采用这种方法分析了所有 10 种草药之后，作者们推断："将这些结果综合在一起表明，就食物过敏疗法要能够全面且持久地抗过敏，并在一定程度上对 Th2/Th1 的免疫反应作出有益改变而言，FAHF-2 所含的草药可能都是必需的。"

"神奇蘑菇"魔力的更多信息

这门科学不必是连续的。尽管临床调查是一步一步小心进行的，以避免对患者造成不必要的伤害，但科学的其他方面，特别是深入研究其影响背后的机制，任何有值得验证的假设和资金的人都可以探究。李秀敏博士研究小组了解到，灵芝中的一些物质可能具有生物活性（比如被称为三萜类的类固醇相关物质），但是哪些物质在灵芝的抗过敏性中发挥着重要作用呢？他们以回顾性标题撰写的《灵芝中的灵芝酸 C1 抑制巨噬细胞和人类外周血单核细胞 TNF-α——通过下调 MAPK、NF-kB 和 AP-1 信号通路而获得的一种产物》

Human Peripheral Blood Mononuclear Cell TNF-α Production by Down-Regulating MAPK, NF-kB and AP-1 Signaling Pathways. "[1]

Noting that *Ganoderma Lucidum* had been used for thousands of years because of its "broad beneficial pharmacological actions," they were particularly drawn to an association with inhibiting production of TNF-α (tumor necrosis factor-alpha). They noted, "TNF-α plays a key role in the immediate host defense against invading microorganisms prior to activation of the adaptive immune system. Excessive levels of TNF-α have been implicated in mediating or exacerbating a number of diseases including Alzheimer's disease, cancer, major depression, and refractory inflammatory diseases including Crohn's disease, rheumatoid arthritis, and asthma."

Dr. Li's team hypothesized that the triterpenes— the compounds in the mushroom that impart a bitter taste—were involved in the inhibition of TNF-α. They have started testing this by first isolating various compounds from *Ling Zhi* and then determining which ones can inhibit TNF-α production by white blood cells isolated from patients with asthma and Crohn's disease (more on TNF-α and Crohn's disease appears in the chapter "Beyond Food Allergies"). Extracts containing mainly triterpenes proved potent inhibitors of TNF-α production by macrophages, the most powerful of which appears to be ganoderic acid C1 (GAC1). The potency also depends on the amount used. It has the advantage of also being nontoxic.

论文(截至写作本书时尚未发表)中探索了这个问题。

值得注意的是,灵芝由于"其广泛而良好的药理学作用",已经应用了数千年,尤其被用到抑制 TNF-α(肿瘤坏死因子-α)产生的组合中。他们指出,"TNF-α 在宿主防御直接抵抗入侵微生物中发挥着关键作用,并且该作用发生在适应免疫系统激活之前。TNF-α 水平过高可能参与介导或加重阿尔茨海默病、癌症和重性抑郁症等大量疾病以及克罗恩病、风湿性关节炎和哮喘等难治的炎症性疾病。"

李秀敏博士研究小组假定三萜类——灵芝中带有苦味的一类化合物——参与抑制 TNF-α。他们已经开始通过从灵芝中分离各种化合物来进行实验,并测定哪些化合物能够通过从哮喘和克罗恩病(关于 TNF-α 和克罗恩病,详见《应用于食物过敏之外的疾病的可能》章节)患者身上分离的白细胞来抑制 TNF-α 的产生。主要包含三萜类的提取物被证明是一种有效的巨噬细胞 TNF-α 抑制剂,其中最有效的成分是灵芝酸 C1(GAC1),其疗效也取决于所用剂

[1] Changda Liu; Nan Yang; Ying Song; Lixin Wang; Jiachen Zi; Bingji Ma; David Dunkin; Keith Benkov; Clare Ceballos; Paula Busse; Jody Tversky; Hugh Sampson; Joseph Goldfarb; Jixun Zhan; Xiu-Min Li., manuscript in preparation.

These results, which mimicked the effects of the whole mushroom extract, lend credence to the team's hypothesis that triterpenes are the active substance.

❽ How Long Does It Last?

Among the food-allergy parents with whom I interact regularly through social media, there are several, for want of a better word, *factions*. One of these consists of mothers who have sought out OIT outside of clinical trials despite the fact that it is not approved for general treatment. OIT is available as part of continuing academic study, which is free, although it often involves considerable expense and travel time to arrive at the participating teaching hospitals. Places in the trials are limited and available only to those who meet certain health criteria. A number of doctors in private practice administer this treatment from protocols that have been proven to their personal satisfaction but are not cleared by the FDA for clinical use. Families usually pay cash, although there are more reports of insurance companies picking up some of the tab, and they often travel hundreds or sometimes thousands of miles to see these doctors.

As a father, I sympathize with parents who are choosing some relief from fear for their children's health even if the outcomes are still unproven to a regulatory standard. Much is unsettled, particularly if the result requires perpetual maintenance dosing. As I can attest to personally, a daily handful of peanuts or Peanut M&Ms sounds better than Grandpa's Lipitor, but I believe that as these mostly very young patients grow up, they will tire of maintenance dosing. Many who grow up under the threat of anaphylaxis to a

量,还具有无毒性的优点。这些结果和灵芝提取物的整体疗效相似,为研究小组的假说(三萜类是其活性物质)提供了支持。

❽ 持续多长时间?

在我经常通过社交媒体与之互动的食物过敏病患的父母中有几个派别,我想不出比派别更好的说法了。其中一个由探索临床试验之外的 OIT 的母亲组成,尽管其未被批准用于一般治疗。作为继续学术研究的一部分,OIT 是免费的,尽管到达参与教学医院通常需要相当大的费用和旅行时间,而且试验地点有限,仅供符合一定健康标准的人们使用。许多私人诊所的医生采用这种治疗方案,该治疗方案已被证明可以达到个人满意程度,但其临床应用并未获得 FDA 的认可。食物过敏家庭通常支付现金,并经常长途跋涉数百甚至数千英里的路程去看医生,尽管有更多的报告说保险公司承担了一些费用。

作为一名父亲,我同情那些为了孩子的健康而选择权宜之计的父母,即使这些方法的结果尚未被证明是否符合监管标准。很多问题还没有解决,特别是如果需要永久维持剂量。尽管我可以证明,每天吃少量花生或 M&Ms 牌花生巧克力豆听起来比爷爷的降胆固醇药要好得多,但是我相信随着年龄的增长,年轻父母会对维持剂量感到厌倦。许多人是在

particular food never develop a taste for it, which means they must continue to find creative ways to take their medicine *forever*. And then there's the common bane of allergic and asthmatic existence, which is to equate absence of symptoms with cure; people who aren't symptomatic for long periods of time get careless. Although it is still too early to say definitively, it seems to me that children who undergo OIT are good candidates to tempt fate as teenagers. Dr. Robert Wood of Johns Hopkins attracted a great deal of attention at the 2013 meeting of the American Academy of Allergy Asthma and Immunology when he announced that desensitization to milk wasn't holding up after 3 to 5 years. He said, "Some of the more dramatic failures had looked like absolute successes in the study. They were tolerating huge amounts of milk; they were about as close to 'cured' as we could imagine."[①] Finally, there is the generic problem of all chronic disease management—patients just stop taking their medicine.

For all these reasons, the prospect of a permanent cure, or at least long-lasting protection, becomes very attractive, which raises the stakes for FAHF-2's success.

We saw in the first phase of Dr. Li's mouse research that protection persisted for as long as 5 weeks past the end of treatment.[②] How much further could it go, and what would it reveal about the mechanisms that produced the improvement? Would its effects go beyond reducing allergies and lead to overall

受某种食物过敏的威胁下长大的,他们决不会对它产生兴趣,这意味着他们必须继续寻找创造性的方法来永远服药。此外,过敏和哮喘共同的可怕之处在于人们将其症状的消失等同于治愈;如果很长时间没有出现症状时,人们就会忽略它。虽然现在下定论还为时尚早,但在我看来,经历OIT 的儿童是挑战命运的青少年的好人选。2013 年,在美国过敏、哮喘及免疫学学会会议上,当约翰·霍普金斯大学的罗伯特·伍德博士宣布,牛奶脱敏三到五年后就会失效,这引起了广泛关注。他说,"在这项研究中,一些更引人注目的失败看起来绝对是成功的。病人耐受着大量的牛奶;他们几乎就像我们所能想象的'被治愈'了。"最后,所有慢性疾病管理都有一个普遍的问题——患者中断服药。

因为这些原因,永久性治愈或至少长期保护的前景就变得非常吸引人,FAHF-2 成功的可能性也增加了。

在李秀敏博士小鼠研究的第一阶段,我们发现治疗结束后的保护作用的持续时间长达五周。它能走得更远吗? 关于产生这种改善的机制,它揭示了什么? 除了减少过敏,它是否会导致免疫系统的整体抑制,这正

①　http://allergicliving.com/index.php/2013/03/13/milk-oral-immunotherapy-not-lasting/.

②　Kamal D S, Jacob D K, Zhong M Z, et al. The Chinese herbal medicine formula FAHF-2 completely blocks anaphylactic reactions in a murine model of peanut allergy[J]. Journal of Allergy and Clinical Immunology, 2005, 115(1): 171 - 178.

suppression of the immune system, which is the problem with oral and injectable corticosteroids? Such corticosteroids reduce inflammation, which can save lives in an emergency (or make it possible for a stricken athlete to return to the lineup), but regular use leaves the body vulnerable to opportunistic infections and other rebound effects. [1]

An unbalanced therapy could create other problems as well, leaving patients vulnerable to attacks from within their own bodies. Could it cause cancer, for example? This was a red flag raised in the early use of the anti-IgE antibody omalizumab, although that has largely been discredited. (Xolair remains, however, painful to pay for and painful to receive and can be allergenic in its own right for some.) And as mentioned, if a treatment reduced IgE but increased IgG excessively, it could result in some form of autoimmune disease.

The desired outcome was immunomodulation. That is, IgE [vil] production would go down but not disappear, and the production of IgG [ood] would increase without taking over completely.

The first experiment with FAHF-2 treatment had shown that tolerance to peanut for 4 weeks after therapy was associated with increased production of the IFN-γ cytokines by CD8$^+$ T cells, which in turn correlates with protection from anaphylaxis.

TGF-β, a protein that controls proliferation, cellular differentiation, and other functions in most

是口服和注射皮质类固醇的问题所在。这种类固醇减少炎症,能够拯救突发事件中的生命(或使患病的运动员有可能恢复运动生涯),但经常使用会使身体容易受到机会性感染和其他反弹效应的影响。

不平衡的治疗还可能造成其他问题,使患者易受到来自人体内部的攻击。例如,它会导致癌症吗?这是早期使用抗 IgE 抗体奥马珠单抗的危险信号,尽管这在很大程度上已经不可信。(但是,奥马珠单抗抗过敏本身也很令人痛苦,而且对一些人来说,它本身会引发过敏症。)如上文所述,如果治疗降低了 IgE 而过度升高了 IgG,则会导致某种形式的自身免疫疾病。

期望的结果是免疫调节。即(坏)IgE 的产生将降低但不会消失,(好)IgG 的产生将增加但不会完全占据免疫系统主导地位。

采用 FAHF-2 治疗的第一个实验显示,治疗后四周的花生耐受性与 CD8$^+$ T 细胞产生的 IFN-γ 细胞因子的增加有关,而这与预防过敏症相关。

TGF-β 蛋白控制大部分细胞的增殖、分化和其他功能,其没有受到影响。

---

[1] http://www.mayo- clinic.com/heal th/steroids/HQO 1431.

cells,[1] was not affected. TGF-β also plays a part in a range of diseases including cancer, allaying concern that recalibrating the immune system in one way might unbalance it in another. There was a slight but significant reduction of IL-10 production as well. These findings suggested that FAHF-2 might have a long-lasting effect and that increased IFN-γ output by CD8[+] T cells may be responsible, but more work was required.

A new study[2] employed the established model of inducing peanut allergy and challenges at intervals of 4 to 10 weeks for a total of 7 challenges over a period of 36 weeks after discontinuation of FAHF-2 treatment. More than any other study I read, this one crystalizes the brilliance of the partnership between ancient medicine and contemporary science. The basic formula was developed by healers who never understood modern chemistry and biology; they just learned what worked through, I suppose, trial and error. Administering it to patients—mice in this case—is really just an extension of that tradition. The results were gratifying; the therapy showed staying power. Wonderful to me, however, is the fact that the observed results can be assayed and quantified. I love it that you can tell time by an old cathedral clock, but it's more fun when you can see the motion of the gears, pendulums, and weights that move the hands.

In this case, treated mice were protected against

TGF-β 在包括癌症的一系列疾病中也起着一定作用,减轻了人们对以一种方式重新校准免疫系统可能导致另一种方式失衡的担忧。同样,IL-10 的产生出现轻微但是值得注意的降低。这些调查结果表明,FAHF-2 可能具有持久的效果,这可能与 CD8[+] T 细胞产生的 IFN-γ 的增加有关,但是需要进行更多的研究工作来证实。

一项新的研究采用已建立的模型诱导和激发花生过敏,在中止 FAHF-2 治疗后 36 周内,进行 7 次激发,间隔 4 ~ 10 周。这项研究比我读到的任何其他研究都更清楚地体现了古代医学和当代科学的完美结合碰撞出的火花。FAHF-2 的基本配方是由没有学过现代医学和生物的中国古代医师研发的;我想,他们只是通过不断试错来学习起作用的东西。将其给予患者——在这项研究中是小鼠——事实上只是传统方法的延伸。结果令人满意,治疗显示出持久效果。但是,令我觉得奇妙的是观测结果能被分析和量化。我喜欢人们可以通过大教堂的钟得知时间,但是当你看见拨动指针的齿轮、钟摆和摆锤移动时,你会觉得更有趣。

在这种情况下,与假治疗组小鼠

① http://en.wikipedia.org/wiki/TGF_beta.
② Kamal D S, Chunfeng Q, Tengfei Z, et al. Food Allergy Herbal Formula-2 silences peanut-induced anaphylaxis for a prolonged posttreatment period via IFN-γ-Producing CD8[+] T cells[J]. Journal of Allergy and Clinical Immunology, 2009, 123(2): 443-451.

anaphylaxis for as long as 36 weeks compared with sham-treated mice. At that juncture, cytokine profiles of splenocytes and MLN cells and found that, even after 36 weeks, the cytokine profiles were similar to those immediately after treatment: increased IFN-γ and reduced Th2 cytokine production. As before, CD8$^+$ T cells from FAHF-2-treated mice showed enhanced IFN- γ production, but there was no increase in the output of CD4$^+$ cells, which, although they "are critical for proper immune cell homeostasis and host defense", can also be "troublemakers" contributing to immune and inflammatory disease.[1] This confirmed expectations that CD8$^+$ is the dominant player and that, once more, the effect of FAHF-2 is to modulate the balance of Th1 and Th2 activity, "curing" one condition without causing another. The hope that a treatment could be administered a few times per year rather than daily or weekly would be a tremendous boon to compliance.

The study showed that a single 7-week course of FAHF-2 treatment prevented anaphylactic reactions for 6 months after therapy, 25% of a mouse's life span, a period that included 6 peanut challenges.

Approximately 9 months after therapy, only 37% of mice showed moderate reactions, whereas all sham-treated mice had severe anaphylaxis symptoms. Serum peanut-specific IgE levels were low throughout the 9-month period, in contrast to anti-IgE treatment, in which free-IgE increased 2 weeks after treatment was discontinued. Blocking antibody IgG2a levels also

相比,治疗小鼠免受过敏症长达36周。脾脏细胞和 MLN 细胞的细胞因子谱显示,36 周后的细胞因子谱与刚完成治疗后的细胞因子谱相似:提高了 IFN-γ 的产生并降低了 Th2 细胞因子的产生。和以前一样,FAHF-2 治疗小鼠的 CD8$^+$T 细胞显示,增加了 IFN-γ 的产生,但是 CD4$^+$ 细胞的产生并未增加,尽管它们"对于合适的免疫细胞内稳态和宿主防御有重要作用",它们仍是免疫和炎性疾病的"麻烦制造者"。这证实了人们的预期,即 CD8$^+$ 细胞是主要的参与者,并且,再次确定 FAHF-2 的作用是调整 Th1 和 Th2 活性之间的平衡,"治愈"一种病症而不引起其他病症。治疗可以每年进行几次而不是每天或每周进行,将更能让患者遵从医嘱。

研究表明,7 周一个疗程的 FAHF-2 治疗可在结束后 6 个月内防止过敏反应,占小鼠寿命的 1/4,其间进行 6 次花生刺激。

治疗后大约 9 个月,只有 37% 的小鼠出现中度反应,而假治疗组所有小鼠出现严重的过敏反应症状。在这 9 个月中,血清花生特异性 IgE 始终保持在低水平,而在抗 IgE 治疗中止后两周,游离 IgE 水平升高。FAHF-2 治疗后,阻断抗体 IgG2a 也

---

① Kiyoshi H, Amanda P, Gol-naz V, et al. Mechanisms underlying helper T-cell plasticity: implications for immune-mediated disease[J]. Journal of Allergy and Clinical Immunology, 2013, 131(5): 1276 - 1287.

remained high after FAHF-2 treatment, thus interfering with mast-cell degranulation by taking up receptor space in a region on the mast cells that in allergic patients is normally dominated by a "high-affinity receptor" known as FceRI.

Thus, in addition to sustained reduction of peanut-specific IgE, increased peanut-specific IgG2a may contribute to the long-term benefits of FAHF-2 treatment by intercepting antigens before they have a chance to do any harm. These results also suggest that FAHF-2 does not induce overall immune suppression but lasting rebalancing of the ratio of IgG [ood] and IgE [vil].

Both *in vivo* and *in vitro* experiments had produced evidence that the herbal formula can produce complete, long-lasting protection against peanut-induced anaphylaxis. The possibility that prolonged protection can be attained without continuous drug treatment represents a significant potential therapeutic advantage over any more conventional or unconventional therapy now envisioned.

❾ Human Trials

▎Contemplating a Human Trial

This research didn't unfold in a straight line. By 2005, though years of research with mice lay ahead, it seemed feasible to the team that FAHF-2 would be proven safe and effective not only for mice but for people, too. The ingredients had been validated by thousands of years of medicinal use. The formula was now adjusted to avoid running afoul of FDA safety standards. Moreover, the effectiveness of the formulas in treating parasites and allergic conditions also pointed toward success.

保持在高水平,并通过占据肥大细胞上的某区域内受体空间而影响肥大细胞脱粒,该区域在过敏患者体内通常由被称为 FceRI 的"高亲和力受体"所支配。

因此,除了花生特异性 IgE 的持续降低,花生特异性 IgG2a 的升高也可能有助于 FAHF-2 在抗原为害之前截取抗原,从而获得长期疗效。这些结果也表明,FAHF-2 没有诱导全身的免疫抑制,而是维持(好)IgG 和(坏)IgE 比值的平衡。

体内实验和体外实验证明,该中药方剂能够产生全面且持久地抵抗花生诱发的过敏反应。不经连续的药物治疗而获得延长的保护作用,这种可能性较预期的传统或非传统治疗方案明显具有潜在的治疗优势。

❾ 人体试验

▎考虑一项人体试验

本研究并非一帆风顺。截至 2005 年,尽管采用小鼠进行了几年相关研究,研究小组似乎不仅能够证明 FAHF-2 对小鼠安全有效,而且对人类同样适用。通过数千年的临床应用,FAHF-2 的成分已得到验证。现在对该配方进行调整,以避免与 FDA 安全标准相冲突。而且,该配方在治疗寄生虫和过敏状况方面的疗效同样指向成功。

The time had come, however, to envision how to formulate the medicines and administer them to people, and in this regard, some of the biggest hurdles weren't regulatory or scientific but cultural.

Chinese herbal preparations are typically boiled and drunk, or boiled, mashed, and combined into pills. The fact that the typical patient in this case would be a child presented an additional challenge. In pill form, WMW is taken for parasites in a regimen of 10 pills 3 times a day before meals; however, this duration is dictated by the lifecycle of the worms, not the years it might take to retrain the immune system for food allergies. For this purpose, it was calculated that 50 pills a day would be required over many months, a dreary prospect for the medical team, so they decided to first try it in liquid form. Yuck! Bitter!

This presented a problem, because substances such as triterpenes in *Ling Zhi* that make them bitter are also the active medicinal components. Dr. Li says that if her colleagues had grown up in China, where large quantities of herbs were drunk from early childhood, they would have had no problem tolerating quantities of bitter tea, but the herbal decoction was unpalatable for Western tastes. Adding sugar only made the bitterness worse. Regardless, home brewing is just a practical impossibility. A one-day therapeutic dose would take approximately 4 ounces of herbs (see chapter 3) with water enough to boil for several hours, and the BTUs it would take to boil them for that long. Multiply that daily regime by 3 to 5 years.

So, pills it was.

然而，设想如何制备药物并将其应用于人类的时代已经到来。就这一点而言，最大的困难不是管理或科学，而是文化。

中草药典型制剂是煮沸饮用，或煮、捣碎并制成药丸。本案例中的典型患者是儿童，这又增加了服药难度。以药丸的形式，服用乌梅丸治疗寄生虫，饭前服用，一天三次，一次10粒；但是，持续服药时间由蛔虫的生命周期所决定，而不是重新训练食物过敏应对免疫系统所需要的几年时间。为此，估算为一天需要50粒药丸，并且持续几个月，对医疗小组而言，前景是黯淡的，所以他们决定首先尝试液体剂型。真难吃！太苦了！

这就存在一个问题，因为灵芝中产生苦味的三萜等物质也是活性药性成分。李秀敏博士说，如果她的同事生长在中国，并且从小就服用大量的草药，那么他们完全可以承受苦味，但是中药汤剂是西方人无法忍受的。加糖也只会让苦味变得更糟。无论如何，在家自制是不切实际的。一天的剂量大约是4盎司草药（见第3章），用足够的水煎煮几个小时，并且煎煮也需要足够的热量。而且，要每天重复这样的操作3到5年。

所以，还是药丸吧。

First Do No Harm

Testing FAHF-2 in human beings has to proceed more judiciously than in the mouse studies. Before testing for FAHF-2's protective effects, the team had to meet the first criterion of any medical therapy—to not make the patient sick in the course of treatment. Mice are rodents. People are people.

The mouse studies had established that FAHF-2 completely blocks peanut-induced anaphylaxis in mice, that mice are protected against anaphylaxis for at least 6 months, and that the effect is associated with sustained suppression of the mechanisms of allergy responses and increased levels of protection. Furthermore, there was a large margin of safety; mice fed 24 times the effective daily dose showed no signs of acute toxic effects, evidence of abnormal liver and kidney functions, abnormal complete blood cell counts, or major organ disease. Human cells tested in the laboratory demonstrated a beneficial immunomodulatory effect of FAHF-2 on peripheral blood mononuclear cells (PBMCs) from children allergic to peanut and at least one other food. These results indicate that FAHF-2 was a candidate to treat a spectrum of the most serious food allergies, not just one at a time. This would make it more useful than allergen-specific OIT, which would take years of desensitizing to one food at a time.

On the basis of the preliminary observations, the team initiated the first-ever phase-1 study to evaluate a treatment for food allergy as an FDA IND botanical drug product (IND 77,468). The drug would be

无损于病人为先

进行人体 FAHF-2 试验,比小鼠试验更要谨慎。在检测 FAHF-2 的保护作用之前,研究小组必须满足药物治疗的第一标准——在治疗过程中,不让患者感到不舒服。小鼠是啮齿动物,而人命关天。

小鼠研究已经确定,FAHF-2 能够完全阻碍小鼠体内花生诱导的过敏性反应,并且可以保护小鼠至少 6 个月不出现过敏反应,这种影响与过敏反应机制的持久抑制和保护水平的增长有关。此外,安全界限很高;用 24 倍的每日有效剂量喂食小鼠,并未显示急性中毒、肝肾功能异常、全血细胞计数异常或重大器官疾病的迹象。实验室中人类细胞的检测表明,FAHF-2 对外周血单核细胞(PBMCs)(来自对花生和至少另外一种食物过敏的儿童)具有良好的免疫调节作用。这些结果表明,FAHF-2 是治疗一系列最严重食物过敏症状的候选药物,不只是一次仅针对一种食物过敏。这让它比过敏原特异性 OIT 更加有用,OIT 花费好多年才一次仅对一种食物脱敏。

在初步观察基础上,研究小组开始进行有史以来第一例第 1 阶段的研究,评估对食物过敏的治疗方法,

given for one week. ① This study was approved by the Mount Sinai Medical Center institutional review board, and each participant provided written informed consent before enrollment.

One major challenge to the integrity of a blinded human trial is for the researchers to remain scrupulously indifferent to anything that might create bias. Dr. Li told me that her friends give her a hard time when she refers to patients in trials as subjects rather than anything more human.

Dr. Julie Wang is one of the physicians who works directly with subjects. She walks a fine line between bedside manner and scientific detachment. She has trained herself not to speculate about whether one subject or another is receiving the drugs or the placebo. It is her job to record any ailment that subjects report, "even a stubbed toe, which obviously has nothing to do with the treatment or the placebo." Wang says that the test subjects often volunteer their own speculation, which the researchers studiously ignore. "During pollen season, they might say, I'm feeling better than I did last year—I must be on FAHF-2, but all I do is to write down their symptoms and forget the rest of it."

Whereas the mouse trials involved only peanut allergy, the first human trial also encompassed tree nuts, fish, and shellfish because after peanut allergies,

并将其作为 FDA IND 植物性药品（IND 77,468）。该药物将服用一周。本研究经西奈山医药中心学会审批委员会批准,各个参与者在录入之前均需提供书面知情同意书。

盲法人体实验完整性的一个主要挑战是研究人员对任何可能导致试验结果出现偏差的事情都要谨慎地保持漠然。李秀敏博士告诉我,当她把试验中的病人看作受试者,而不是生活中的人时,她的朋友对她有很多怨言。

朱莉·王博士是直接与受试者打交道的医生之一。在医生对待患者应有的同情关切的态度和客观严谨的科学态度之间,她把握的很小心。她训练自己不去推测一个人是在服用药物还是安慰剂。她的工作就是记录受试者所述的病痛,"甚至脚趾骨折,这明显与治疗或安慰剂无关。"王博士说,受测者经常主动提出自己的猜测,而研究人员要故意忽略这些推测。"在花粉季节,他们可能会说感觉比去年好多了——自己一定是在使用 FAHF-2,而我能做的就是记录他们的症状,忽略其他事情。"

但是,小鼠实验仅涉及了花生过敏,首次人体试验也包括坚果、鱼和贝类,因为在花生过敏之后,对这些

---

① Julie W, Sangita P P, Nan Y, et al. Safety, tolerability, and immunologic effects of a food allergy herbal formula in food allergic individuals: a randomized, double-blinded, placebo-controlled, dose escalation, phase 1 study [J]. Annals of Allergy, Asthma & Immunology, 2010, 105(1): 75-84.

allergies to these are least likely to be outgrown. Individuals aged 12 through 45 years of age were eligible. Their history of these allergies was documented by positive skin-test results and/or food allergen-specific IgE level. Females of childbearing potential had to either be sexually inactive or using effective birth-control measures for the duration of the study.

Candidates were excluded for acute infection; history of systemic diseases; abnormal hepatic, bone marrow, or renal function; clinically significant abnormal electrocardiogram result; current uncontrolled moderate-to-severe asthma; drug or alcohol abuse; pregnancy or lactation; and participation in another research protocol within the previous 30 days.

This was a randomized, double-blind, placebo-controlled (neither researchers nor subjects knew who was getting FAHF-2 or placebo), dose-escalation, phase-1 trial three doses of FAHF-2 were used: 2. 2 grams (4 tablets), 3. 3 grams (6 tablets), and 6. 6 grams (12 tablets) 3 times a day for 7days—a dose range based on previous experience with FAHF-2 in animal models. Four active and 2 placebo patients were treated at each level, and doses were increased after independent review of the data from the 6 patients receiving the lower dose.

Initial evaluation consisted of a thorough medical history and physical examination, vital signs, skin-prick testing and food-specific IgE testing, baseline pulmonary function, electrocardiography, urinalysis, and routine laboratory blood tests (complete blood cell count, serum chemical analyses, renal function, liver function tests, and pregnancy test for female

过敏的可能性最小。受试者的年龄区间为 12～45 岁。他们的过敏史以阳性皮肤检测结果以及/或食物过敏特异性 IgE 水平记录在案。在研究期间,具有生育能力的女性必须性生活不活跃,或者使用有效的节育措施。

以下人群不能参与实验:有急性感染;有系统性疾病史;肝、骨髓或肾功能异常;临床心电图明显异常;目前未得到控制的中、重度哮喘;滥用药物或酒精;怀孕或哺乳期妇女;过去 30 天内参与了其他研究治疗方案。

本实验是随机双盲安慰剂对照(研究人员和受试者都不知道谁正在服用 FAHF-2 或安慰剂)实验,增加剂量,第 1 阶段实验使用三种剂量的 FAHF-2:2.2 克(4 片)、3.3 克(6 片)和 6.6 克(12 片),每天 3 次,连续 7 天——这个剂量范围是基于前期动物模型所采用 FAHF-2 的经验。在每种剂量上治疗 4 例活动期患者和 2 例服用安慰剂的患者,并在单独观察 6 名接受低剂量患者的数据之后,增加给药剂量。

初步评估包括一份详尽病史和体检、生命体征、皮肤点刺试验和食物特异性 IgE 试验、基础肺功能、心电图、尿液分析以及实验室血常规检查(全血细胞计数、血清化学分析、肾功能、肝功能检查和女性参与者的妊娠测试)。

participants).

After initial screening, patients were prescribed either FAHF-2 or placebo for 7 days. Patients continued food-allergen avoidance for the duration of the study and were asked to refrain from other herbal medication use. Investigators spoke twice with each patient by telephone during the 7-day period to reinforce medication compliance and assess potential adverse effects. Patients were instructed to complete a symptom diary. During the final visit, the medical history was reviewed again and a final physical examination was done, including spirometry, a measurement of lung function, specifically the volume and/or speed of air that can be inhaled and exhaled. This is used to assess asthma severity. Electrocardiography and laboratory testing were also done.

Before enrollment and at the end of the week-long treatment, titrated SPTs were performed with stock peanut or individual tree nut, fish, and/or shellfish extracts, as well as negative saline controls and positive controls using a histamine base. Levels of interleukins, IFN-γ, and other pertinent cytokines were measured throughout using some of the laboratory methods described in previous chapters.

A total of 23 patients with food allergy underwent initial evaluation. Of these, 2 were excluded who had no evidence of food allergy on skin-prick testing and serum specific IgE testing, and 2 had uncontrolled asthma. No clinically significant differences were found between the FAHF-2 and placebo groups at baseline.

Nineteen patients were enrolled and randomized to FAHF-2 or placebo treatments; 1 patient withdrew

初步筛选后,患者持续服用 FAHF-2 或安慰剂 7 天。在研究中,患者继续回避食物过敏原,并避免服用其他草药。在这 7 天,调查员每天与各个患者通话两次,以便加强服药依从性,评估潜在副作用。患者在指导下填写症状日志。在最后一次回访时,再次评估病史,进行最后一次身体检查,包括肺活量测定,这是一项肺功能检测,尤其是肺部吸入和呼出空气的体积和速度,用于评估哮喘的严重程度。然后,进行心电图和实验室检测。

在入组前和为期一周的治疗最后,采用普通花生或个别坚果、鱼和/或贝类提取物,以及阴性生理盐水对照和阳性组胺对照进行皮肤点刺试验的滴定。采用之前章节中所描述的一些实验室方法测量白介素、IFN-γ 和其他相关细胞因子的含量。

对 23 例食物过敏患者进行了初步评估。其中,排除 2 例在皮肤刺痛测试中未出现食物过敏反应的患者,还有 2 例患有不受控制的哮喘。基线期内,FAHF-2 和安慰剂组之间未发现临床显著差异。

19 例患者入选并随机接受 FAHF-2 或安慰剂治疗;第二天(第 6

from the study after the second day（sixth dose）because of an allergic reaction. Eighteen patients（12 patients in the FAHF-2 group and 6 in the placebo group）successfully completed 7 days of treatment and were included in the analyses evaluating the tolerability and safety of FAHF-2.

Escalation was allowed in a group if none of the 6 experienced a toxic effect as defined by a grade-3 adverse event（AE）attributable to the medication. The standards were adapted from the World Health Organization（WHO）standards, except that they were applied more stringently. A grade-1 "mild" AE according to the WHO was regarded as a grade-3 "severe" event for purposes of this study. If 1 of 6 patients in the FAHF-2 group had experienced such a toxic effect, then 6 additional patients（again, 4 in the FAHF-2 group and 2 in the placebo group）were added to that group and the dose escalation delayed until the additional patients completed the safety evaluation. If fewer than 2 of the 12 patients in the group experienced a dose-limiting toxic effect, the next 6 were enrolled at a higher dose. If 2 of the 12 patients experienced a dose-limiting toxic effect on any specified dose, no additional patients were to be enrolled at that dose or higher dose, pending further discussions with the independent safety reviewers.

No grade-3 AEs occurred in patients treated with FAHF-2. One patient receiving the drug reported diffuse urticaria—hives—3 hours after the sixth dose（12 tablets）, but no other associated symptoms. He was instructed to stop using the study medication. The rash progressively worsened, and he was seen in a local emergency department 24 hours later. Physical

次服药）后,1 例患者因为过敏反应而退出本研究。18 例患者（12 例患者在 FAHF-2 组,6 例患者在安慰剂组）成功完成了 7 天的治疗,并被纳入评估 FAHF-2 的耐受性和安全性的分析中。

如果 6 例患者均未出现定义为由药物引起的 3 级不良事件（AE）的毒性作用,则允许增加药量。本标准改编自世界卫生组织（WHO）标准,只是应用起来更加严格。在本研究中,根据 WHO 设定的 1 级"轻度"不良事件,被视为 3 级"严重"事件。如果 FAHF-2 组有 1/6 患者出现这种毒性作用,则增加 6 例患者（FAHF-2 组增加 4 例,安慰剂组增加 2 例）,并且剂量增加延迟,直到新增加的患者完成安全评估。如果实验组患者少于 2 例表现出剂量限制毒性作用,则给予其他 6 例高剂量药物。如果 12 例患者中有 2 例对某一剂量表现出剂量限制性毒性,则不再对其他患者进行该剂量或更高剂量的药物治疗,有待与独立安全评审人进一步讨论。

FAHF-2 治疗的患者并未出现 3 级 AEs。一名接受该药治疗的患者报告说,在第六次服药（12 片）3 小时后出现了风疹——荨麻疹,但是无其他相关症状。他被告知停止服用该研究药物。皮疹逐渐恶化 24 小时后,他在当地急诊室接受了治疗。皮

examination and treatment by a dermatologist indicated this was a flare-up of atopic dermatitis unrelated to the study. The patient returned for skin-prick testing with FAHF-2 one month later, which was negative, but he had a reaction to the positive control (histamine) and no reaction to the negative control (saline); therefore, this reaction was deemed unlikely to be related to the study medication.

Of the 18 participants who completed 7 days of treatment, 1 FAHF-treated patient out of 12 (8%) reported loose bowel movements once a day on days 1 through 4, which normalized thereafter, and 1 placebo-treated patient out of 6 (17%) reported a single episode of vomiting on day 4. Neither patient required treatment.

Overall, no significant differences were found in laboratory values obtained at baseline or after completing FAHF-2 treatment. Pulmonary-function tests and electrocardiogram findings before and after treatment remained substantially constant, as did allergen-specific IgE and SPT results before and after 7 days of FAHF-2 treatment. *In vitro* treatment of patients' PBMCs with FAHF-2 showed reduced IL-5 secretion and increased IFN-g and IL-10 secretion. The conclusion: FAHF-2 is safe and well tolerated in food-allergic patients.

Extended Phase-1 Study—Inhibiting Effect on Basophils[①]

The original 7-day study was encouraging for its

肤科医生进行的体检和治疗表明,这是与本研究不相关的急性异位皮肤炎。一个月之后,采用 FAHF-2 对该患者进行皮肤点刺试验,结果呈阴性,但是他对阳性对照(组胺)有反应,而对阴性对照(生理盐水)无反应;因此,认为该反应不太可能与本研究药物有关。

在完成 7 天治疗的 18 例患者中,FAHF 组 12 例患者中有 1 例患者(8%),从第 1 天至第 4 天每天腹泻一次,之后正常;安慰剂组 6 例患者中有 1 例患者(17%)在第 4 天出现呕吐症状。均不需要治疗。

总之,在基线期内或完成 FAHF-2 治疗后获得的实验室数值均未发现明显差异。治疗前后,肺功能检测和心电图检测结果基本保持一致,为期 7 天的 FAHF-2 治疗前后的过敏原特异 IgE 和 SPT 结果同样也保持不变。对外周血单核细胞进行 FAHF-2 体外处理,显示 IL-5 分泌降低以及 IFN-g 和 IL-10 分泌升高。结论是在治疗食物过敏患者过程中,FAHF-2 安全并且耐受性良好。

第 1 阶段研究延伸——对嗜碱性粒细胞的抑制作用

最初为期 7 天的研究因其安全

---

① Sangita P P, Julie W, Ying S, et al. Clinical safety of Food Allergy Herbal Formula-2 (FAHF-2) and inhibitory effect on basophils from patients with food allergy: extended phase I study. [J] Journal of Allergy and Clinical Immunology, 2011, 128(6): 1259－1265.

safety and tolerability and because underlying cellular activity pointed to favorable effects on the immune system, consistent with those from the mouse trials. It was a double-blind, placebo-controlled clinical trial, the "gold standard" because neither patients nor researchers know which subjects are getting a placebo and which ones are getting the treatment. Because subjects don't know, their beliefs and expectations don't taint the results. Because the researchers don't know either, they can't inadvertently hint to patients about what to expect and what the results will be.

A second phase-1 study was designed to evaluate safety and tolerability over a longer period of time, with additional study of physiological changes without the poking, prodding, force-feeding, blood-letting, hazardous food challenges, and, of course, dissection that can be done on mice.

Unlike the first trial, however, this was an open-label study. Each participant would receive the medication. Convinced now that FAHF-2 works (i. e. , is safe and influences the underlying biochemistry in a favorable direction), Dr. Li and her colleagues wanted to study its effects on a broad set of measures. Because they couldn't regularly challenge their subjects as they had the mice, however, the researchers needed to find a biomarker that could be studied in the laboratory and dosed with antigens without risking anyone's health.

They chose the basophil. Basophils comprise less than 1% of leukocytes, but, like mast cells, are critical to allergic reactions, especially the later phases

性和耐受性而令人鼓舞,因为基础细胞活性表明对免疫系统有良好影响,这与小鼠试验的结果一致。本次实验是双盲的安慰剂对照临床试验,即"黄金标准",无论是患者还是研究人员,均不知道哪些受试者服用安慰剂,哪些受试者服用药物。因为受试者不知道,所以他们的想法和期望就不会影响实验结果。因为研究人员也不知道,所以他们不会因为疏忽而暗示患者预期怎样以及结果是什么。

第 1 阶段的第二次研究旨在为评估更长时间内的安全性和耐受性,并对生理变化进行额外研究,而无须针刺、强制喂食、放血、危险食物激发,当然还有小鼠实验中的解剖。

但是,与第一次实验不同,这次是非盲试验。各个参与者均会服用药物。经确认,FAHF-2 是有效的(即,它是安全的,并以有利的方向影响潜在的生物化学),李秀敏博士和她的同事想要研究其对一系列措施的影响。因为他们不能像刺激小鼠那样定期刺激受试者,然而,研究人员需要找到一种生物标记物,让他们可以在实验室进行研究,并在不危及任何人健康的情况下使用抗原。

他们选择了嗜碱性粒细胞。嗜碱性粒细胞包含不到1%的白细胞,但是,就像肥大细胞一样,它们对于过敏

because by circulating, they provide "reinforcements" to a defense that is already underway. Unlike mast cells, which are lodged in tissue, basophils can be extracted from the blood.

The basophil-activation test (BAT) requires very small quantities of blood and does not require isolation of cells. The case for using basophils as a biomarker was buttressed by another study by Jones et al[1] showing that basophil activation was significantly reduced by 4 to 6 months of OIT and that inhibition of basophils correlated with clinical protection irrespective of IgE levels. In other words, the dogs wouldn't bark or bite every time someone knocked on the front door.

Potential subjects were screened for the same criteria listed above. In the study, participants were started on FAHF-2 (3. 3 g, 6 tablets) 3 times a day for 6 months. They continued to avoid their food allergens for the duration of the study and were asked to refrain from other herbal medication use. Study investigators telephoned every other week to reinforce and confirm medication compliance and to assess potential AEs, and saw subjects every 8 weeks. As before, all participants were instructed to complete a symptom diary. At each visit, the interim medical history was reviewed, and physical examination, spirometry, electrocardiography, and laboratory studies were repeated. Although this study did not include a control group of untreated subjects, as discussed, evidence from other research suggests what a control

反应是很重要的,尤其是后期通过循环,它们能向进行中的防御保护提供"补给"。不像肥大细胞寄宿在组织中,嗜碱性粒细胞可以从血液中提取。

嗜碱性粒细胞激活试验(BAT)需要少量的血液,并且不要求分离细胞。采用嗜碱性粒细胞作为生物标记物的理由得到了琼斯等人的另一项研究的支持,表明进行4~6个月OIT后,嗜碱性粒细胞活性显著降低,嗜碱性粒细胞的抑制与临床保护相关而与IgE水平无关。换句话说,狗不会在每次有人敲门时都吠叫或咬人。

采用前述标准对潜在的参与者进行筛选。在本研究中,受试者服用FAHF-2(3.3克,6片),每天3次,共服用6个月。在研究期间,他们继续回避食物过敏原,并按要求避免服用其他草药。研究调查员每隔一周对受试者进行电话回访,加强并确定服药依从性以及评估潜在不良事件,每8周观察受试者一次。如以前那样,参与者在指导下填写症状日志。每次回访都会审查临时病历,重复体检、肺活量测定、心电图以及实验室研究。但正如之前讨论过的,其他研究所显示的证据已经表明在有对照组的情况下会产生的结果。琼斯等人报告,在这6个月中,仅仅避免花生诱导并"没有"降低嗜碱性粒细胞的激活反应。此外,参与西奈山研究的大部分

① Jones S M, Pons L, Roberts J L, et al. Clinical efficacy and immune regulation with peanut oral immunotherapy [J]. Journal of Allergy and Clinical Immunology, 2009, 124(2): 292 - 300.

group might have produced. Jones et al reported that merely avoiding peanut for 6 months *does not* reduce basophil-activation responses. Like most diagnosed food-allergy patients, moreover, most of the patients in the Sinai study had avoided their food allergens for several years before enrolling in the study and yet their blood showed a high baseline level of basophil activation when exposed to antigens in the test tube. [1]

Studies like this are critically dependent on a consistently high-quality source of test material. The FAHF-2 used came from the same high-quality batch from the acute phase-1 study. An HPLC fingerprint of FAHF-2 was generated by Dr. Yang's team with an eye to standardizing the FAHF-2 product and to monitoring consistency and shelf life. This fingerprint helped establish the consistency of FAHF-2 used during both the phase-1 trial in July 2007 and the second study a year later.

Eighteen subjects were enrolled, but 4 withdrew: 1 because of pregnancy, 2 because of the time required and high number of tablets taken daily, and 1 with transient abdominal complaints without vomiting or diarrhea.

The median age of the patients was 16 years (range 12 – 27 years), and 2/3 were male. No patient was allergic only to peanut, and all but 5% had other allergic diseases, including asthma, allergic rhinitis, and atopic dermatitis.

患者正如大部分确诊的食物过敏患者一样,在入组之前,已经好几年没有接触过食物过敏原,然而当其血液接触试管中的抗原时,血液表现为高基准水平的嗜碱性粒细胞活性。

此类研究非常依赖始终如一的高质量测试材料来源。所使用的FAHF-2来自急性第1阶段研究所用的同一批次优质材料。FAHF-2的HPLC指纹图谱由杨博士的团队生成,目的是标准化FAHF-2产品并监控一致性和保质期。这个指纹图谱帮助建立了所使用的FAHF-2在2007年7月的阶段1试验和一年后的第二次试验中的一致性。

共纳入18例受试者,但是4例退出:1例因为怀孕而退出,2例因为时间不允许和每天服用大量药片而退出,1例出现短暂的腹部不适,无呕吐或腹泻现象。

患者的中位年龄是16岁(12～27岁),其中2/3是男性患者。没有患者只对花生过敏,5%患有其他过敏疾病,包括哮喘、过敏性鼻炎和异位性皮肤炎。

---

[1] There is a misconception, promulgated even by some allergists according to reports I have gotten, that strict avoidance can make the body "forget" that it is allergic. Some people do "outgrow" their allergies, for reasons not fully understood, but "forgetting" probably has nothing to do with it.

根据我得到的报告,存在一种误解,甚至一些过敏症专家也宣扬了这种误解,即严格的禁忌(某些食物)会让身体"忘记"它是致敏的。有些人确实"长大了",不再过敏,原因还不完全清楚,但"忘记"可能与此无关。

There were no changes in hematology or chemistry laboratory values, pulmonary function, or electrocardiographic findings obtained at baseline, at 2-month intervals, or after completion of 6 months of FAHF-2 treatment. Neither were there changes in SPTs at baseline or after 6 months of FAHF-2 treatment.

One patient had an AE. She had a previous history of EoE (a form of allergic inflammation caused when white blood cells called eosinophils infiltrate the esophagus, where they don't normally appear), which had been diagnosed two years before but was not believed to have active disease and was not receiving treatment when the study began. After 5 1/2 weeks on FAHF-2 treatment, she contacted the study coordinator to report that she had what she believed to be a recurrence of her EoE. She was instructed to discontinue FAHF-2 until her gastroenterologist could evaluate her. The gastroenterologist performed an upper endoscopy, which did reveal inflammation. After treatment for her gastric problems, the participant was restarted on FAHF-2 and completed the study with no other abdominal complaints.

BATs were performed on the blood of the other 11 patients. These tests monitor basophil expression of the protein CD63 on the cell surface. They showed a significant reduction in basophil percentages after 6 months of FAHF-2 treatment when challenged in test tubes.

These results not only suggest that long-term use of FAHF-2 safe, but also provide strong evidence that FAHF-2 may be effective in treating food allergy. As always, additional studies were needed.

在基线期、每隔 2 个月或完成 FAHF-2 治疗 6 个月后获得的血液学或化学实验室值、肺功能或心电图结果没有变化。在基线期或 FAHF-2 治疗 6 个月后，皮肤点刺试验也没有变化。

有一例患者发生不良事件。她有 EoE（嗜酸性粒细胞性食管炎，被称为嗜酸性粒细胞的白细胞渗入食道后从而引起过敏炎症，这种白细胞通常不会出现在食道）病史，是在两年前确诊的，但不被认为是活动期疾病。当研究开始时，她也没有接受治疗。进行 FAHF-2 治疗五周半后，她联系研究协调员说，她认为自己的 EoE 复发了。协调员指示她停止服用 FAHF-2，直到她的胃肠病医师对她进行评估为止。胃肠病医师对她进行了胃镜检查，结果显示有炎症。对胃病进行治疗后，她又重新开始服用 FAHF-2 并完成了研究，且期间没有出现其他腹部疾病。

对其他 11 例患者的血液进行了嗜碱性粒细胞激活试验。这些实验检测了细胞表面的蛋白质 CD63 的嗜碱性粒细胞表达。结果显示，在试管中进行 6 个月的 FAHF-2 治疗后，嗜碱性粒细胞比例显著下降。

这些结果不仅表明长期使用 FAHF-2 是安全的，而且为 FAHF-2 可能有效治疗食物过敏提供了有力证据。像往常一样，还需要进一步研究。

❿ Too Many Pills

As mentioned earlier, one of the biggest obstacles to controlling chronic disease according to medical professionals of all credentials—doctors, nurses, and pharmacists alike—is getting patients to follow their prescribed treatment—so-called compliance, or adherence. This is certainly the case with asthma. Patients often don't take their inhaled medication twice a day, as instructed, or monitor their peak flows as often as they should. They are also advised to avoid the things that trigger their disease to the greatest extent possible, but can't, or don't.

Because there is no preemptive medication for food allergies, patients are stuck with avoiding their offending foods as their sole day-to-day strategy, which has frustrations of its own. When the child is an infant and toddler, parents have a big say in his or her daily activities and eating habits. By the age of three or four, most children under the care of a conscientious doctor and diligent parents can begin to take part in their own avoidance. Many children learn to read labels very young and will alert a parent when there is danger.

At these ages, one of the greatest threats is from caregivers. One study shows that 11% of anaphylaxis incidents result from parents, babysitters, grandparents, and others feeding children the food intentionally.[①] Another study at Johns Hopkins listed a number of rationales by parents for giving a child a forbidden

❿ 药丸数量太多

如前所述,根据拥有各种资历的医疗人员(医生、护士和药剂师等)所说,控制慢性疾病的最大障碍之一是让患者遵循指定的治疗,即所谓的依从性或坚持。哮喘就是这样。患者经常不遵循一天服用2次药物的医嘱,或没有尽可能频繁地监测自己的峰值。按建议他们应尽可能避免接触能诱导他们自身疾病的物质,但是他们不能避免或不注意避免这些物质。

因为没有药物可以预防食物过敏,所以患者将避免接触引起过敏的食物作为唯一的日常策略。孩子在婴儿期或学步期间,父母在其日常活动和饮食习惯中扮演重要角色。到三四岁时,在有责任心的医生和勤勉的父母的照顾下,大多数儿童自己能够主动避免食用令其过敏的食物。许多儿童在很小时候就学会看标签,当有危险时会警告父母。

在这几个年龄段,最大的威胁之一来自看护者。一项研究显示,11%的过敏事件是由父母、保姆、祖父母以及其他故意喂孩子过敏食物的人造成的。约翰·霍普金斯大学的另一项研究列举了父母给孩子吃被禁

① http://www. sciencedaily. com/ releases/2012/06/120625125952. htm？ utm ＿ source ＝ feedburner&utm ＿＿ medium ＝ email&utm_campaign ＝ Fee d％ 3 A ＋ sciencedaily％ 2Fhealth_medicine％ 2Fallergy ＋ ％ 28Science Daily ％ 3 A ＋ Health ＋ ％ 2 6 ＋ Medicine ＋ Newsn— ＋ Allergy％ 29.

food, among them that they didn't believe small exposures would provoke a reaction, to see if the allergy had resolved, as "do-it-yourself immunotherapy," or that they didn't believe the diagnosis. Teenagers sometimes try forbidden foods deliberately. Then, too, only 27% of patients who experience anaphylaxis are given an epinephrine auto-injector, the most effective emergency treatment.[1] Many patients and caregivers hesitate to use epinephrine because they are fearful of side effects, especially the jolt it may give to a young heart. The conventional wisdom, however, is that epinephrine represents no threat to the child's health, especially compared to the potential for tragedy from a wait-and-see approach.

If OIT proves itself as a mainstream therapy, adherence will become an issue, although it may entail a handful of peanut M&Ms rather than a couple of puffs on an inhaler. A cure would be better.

As mentioned in chapter 8, Dr. Li and her colleagues decided early on that FAHF-2 should be delivered in pill form rather than as a decoction, or tea. "Liquid works with Chinese children who are used to drinking medicinal tea from a very young age," says Dr. Li, "for the weeks it takes to treat intestinal parasites." To "reeducate" the immune system—Dr. Li's word, not mine—and cure food allergies over many months or even years is another matter.

But how many pills? Evaporating the unrefined decoction produced a daily dose of 50 pills. This was

止的食物的一些案例的原因,有些父母不相信轻微接触会引起过敏反应,为了看过敏是否已被解决或不相信诊断,会按照"自己动手的免疫疗法"给孩子吃少量被禁止的食物。有时候,青少年会故意尝试被禁止的食物。然后,只有27%的过敏患者会被注射肾上腺素,而这是最有效的紧急治疗方法。许多患者和看护者不愿使用肾上腺素,因为他们害怕副作用,尤其是心脏震颤的副作用。然而,传统观点认为肾上腺素不会对孩子的健康构成威胁,尤其是与采取观望态度可能导致的悲剧相比。

如果证明 OIT 是主流疗法,则依附性会变成一个问题,尽管它可能需要一把 M&Ms 花生巧克力豆,而不是在吸入器上喷几口。有治愈疗法当然更好了。

如第8篇所述,李秀敏博士和她的同事很早就决定,FAHF-2 应以药丸形式而非汤剂或茶的形式开出。"汤剂对从很小就开始喝药茶的中国儿童行得通,"她说,"它要花费几周时间治疗肠道寄生虫。""而花费几个月甚至几年'再教育'免疫系统(这是李秀敏博士说的,不是我说的)治疗食物过敏与之大相径庭。"

但是,服用多少药丸呢?将未提炼的汤剂蒸发制成药丸,每日剂量

---

① http://allergicliving.com/index.php/2012/04/2 7/ time-to-end-food-allergy-tragedies/? page=2.

reduced to 36 for the 6-month extension of the phase-1 human trial, during which 2 of the 18 participants aged 12 to 45 dropped out because of compliance issues. Part of the problem was the time commitment involved, but the number of pills was also a factor. Unless the number could be reduced, FAHF-2 would never become a useful mass treatment. Life in food-allergy families is already stressful. The prospect of standing over a child 3 times a day to make him take 12 pills for years on end is daunting.

Water extraction was the logical first step because it mixes so well with so many things. It is the "universal solvent." In the right concentrations, salt, sugar, and many other things can remain dissolved in water indefinitely. Water has its limits for separating the active ingredients in FAHF-2 from unnecessary residues from the original herbs, however.

The way forward was to make a more concentrated pill. If more of the active ingredients could be contained in a pill of the same volume and weight, then fewer of them would be necessary. How were they to do this? Scientists resort to complicated schemes based on how easily different compounds dissolve in different liquids. The idea is to remove as many impurities and inert residues from the compounds you are interested in as possible. Although the new pills may be chemically identical, however, the new formulations still must be tested for effectiveness (the purification could mangle the compounds) and safety.

Water by itself couldn't remove the impurities. However, using ethanol, which is less polar than

50 粒。因为第 1 阶段人体实验延长 6 个月，所以每日剂量降至 36 粒，在此期间，12～45 岁的 18 例受试者中，有 2 例因为依从性问题而退出。一方面原因就是所涉及的时间投入，但是药丸剂量也是一个原因。除非药丸剂量降低，否则 FAHF-2 就不能在大规模群体中推广使用。在有食物过敏病人的家庭中，生活压力已经很大。每天监督一个儿童每日服用 3 次药丸，每次 12 粒，连续服用几年，这样的前景令人生畏。

水提取液在逻辑上是第一步，因为它能很好地与很多东西混合，是"通用的溶剂"。在合适的浓度中，盐、糖以及其他物质成分能够永远地溶解在水中。然而，要从原始草药的剩余残渣中分离 FAHF-2 的活性成分，水也有一定的局限性。

因此，研究的方向就是制备更浓缩的药丸。如果相同体积相同重量的一颗药丸能够包含更多的活性成分，则所需剂量就会更少。如何才能实现呢？科学家采用了复杂的方案，该方案是基于不同化合物在不同液体中溶解的难易程度。该方法就是尽可能多地除去化合物中的杂质和无效残渣。尽管新药丸的化学成分可能完全一样，但是新配方的疗效（提纯可能会损坏化合物的结构）和安全性仍需要检测。

水本身不能除去杂质，但是采用极性比水小的乙醇就可以进一步提

water, they were able to further extract the active ingredients in FAHF-2 cutting the daily dose by approximately 30% while retaining efficacy and safety. Reducing a daily dose of 36 pills by 30% still leaves us with a massive number of pills to be taken at each meal, however. Dr. Li's team then used a solvent that is even less polar than ethanol: butanol.

Based on the known characteristics of FAHF-2, the team hypothesized that the less-polar solvent butanol would retain even more of the active compounds. Because butanol isn't also soluble with water, it can be separated from water and the medicinal compounds that dissolve better in butanol are attracted to that layer. Picture salad dressing made of oil, vinegar, and herbs. When the oil rises to the top, the heavier vinegar sinks to the bottom and takes the herbs with it, while the oil remains clear, although in this case, the lighter butanol would rise to the top with the active ingredients while the impurities would remain in the heavier aqueous (water) layer.

Powdered FAHF-2 extract was dissolved in distilled water and dispersed with ultrasound waves for 15 minutes, in which an electrical signal is converted into a physical vibration (called sonification), helping break apart compounds or cells. The aqueous layer was extracted with butanol 4 times in all. Each time, more of the inert residue was removed and the active ingredients became more concentrated. Drying them so they could be shaped into pills presented one additional challenge. Because butanol has a high boiling point compared to water (118 ℃ vs. 100 ℃), drying would take longer, which would become a problem especially after manufacturing is scaled up. Prolonged exposure

取 FAHF-2 的活性成分,从而使每日剂量降低约30%,同时可保证疗效和安全性。然而,即使每日剂量(36粒)降低30%,每次剂量仍然很大。因此,李秀敏博士研究小组采用了一种极性甚至比乙醇还小的溶剂,即丁醇。

结合已知的 FAHF-2 特性,研究小组假设,极性更小的溶剂丁醇将保留更多的活性化合物。因为丁醇不溶于水,所以它可以与水分离,而易溶于丁醇的药用化合物被带到丁醇层。想象一下用油、醋和草药做成的沙拉酱。当油上升到顶部时,较重的醋会带着草药下沉到底部,而上层的油仍然是透明的。然而在这个实验里,较轻的丁醇会带着活性成分上升到顶部,而杂质将留在较重的含水(水)层中。

将粉末状的 FAHF-2 提取物溶于蒸馏水中,然后用超声波分散15分钟,在此期间,电信号被转化成物理振动(称为超声处理)以帮助分解化合物或细胞。采用丁醇将水层提纯4次。每次都会除去很多无效残渣,而活性成分含量也变得更高。然而将活性成分干燥至能制成药丸又是另外一项挑战。因为丁醇的沸点比水高(118 ℃:100 ℃),所以干燥需要更长的时间,这将成为一个问题,尤其是扩大生产之后。长时间的

to higher heat might also "overcook" the ingredients. Ethanol's boiling point, by contrast, is only 79° C, which is why when you cook with wine or brandy, you can get rid of the alcohol without losing the flavor. The solution was to add water to the butanol, which lowered the boiling point. The combined butanol extracts of concentrated active compounds were then mixed with distilled water at a 3-to-1 ratio and evaporated under reduced pressure.

Would It Work?

It remained to be seen whether the new extract would be as potent as the less-refined versions.

After inducing peanut allergy as before, mice were treated with the new medicine, dubbed B-FAHF-2, at a dose only 1/5 by volume as had been used previously, with sham-treated mice as controls.[①] Blood was collected at the time of each challenge, and body temperatures were recorded.

B-FAHF-2 produced prolonged protection against anaphylaxis despite multiple peanut challenges. By the sixth and seventh challenges, at week 40 and 50 after the first course of therapy, half the treated mice developed score-2 mild reactions to the periodic challenges with peanut allergen. Thus, even after almost a full year, the median scores of B-FAHF-2-treated mice were significantly lower than sham-treated mice.

A second course of B-FAHF-2 treatment 8 1/2 months after the first course of treatment restored complete protection against the final challenge at week

高温加热可能会使成分被煮过头。解决方法是在丁醇中加水,这样可以降低沸点。然后将丁醇浓缩活性化合物的组合提取物与蒸馏水以3:1的比例混合,减压蒸发。相比而言,乙醇的沸点只有79℃,这也是为什么用葡萄酒或白兰地做饭时,我们能够除去酒精而不失酒香的原因。

是否可行?

新提取物是否和提纯前提取物有同样疗效,还有待观察。

像以前一样诱导花生过敏之后,给小鼠服用被称为 B-FAHF-2 的新药丸,采用之前剂量的1/5,假治疗组小鼠作为对照。每次刺激时,采集血样并记录体温。

尽管进行了多次花生刺激,B-FAHF-2 还是产生了长效抗过敏性。到第一个疗程后,第40周第6次和第50周的第7次刺激为止,1/2 的小鼠对花生过敏原的定期诱导出现了2级轻度反应。因此,甚至几乎一整年之后,服用 B-FAHF-2 的小鼠的中位得分仍显著低于假治疗组小鼠。

第一个疗程八个半月后,采用 B-FAHF-2 治疗的第二个疗程在第65周恢复了对最后刺激的抵抗。因

---

① Srivastava K, Yang N, Chen Y, et al. Efficacy, safety and immunological actions of butanol-extracted Food Allergy Herbal Formula-2 on peanut anaphylaxis[J]. Clinical & Experimental Allergy, 2011, 41(4): 582 – 591.

65. Mice were therefore significantly protected for approximately 12 months, half of their life span. Protection was registered by the now-familiar clinical measures as well as by observed signs of anaphylaxis. Peanut-allergic sham-treated mice had significantly lower body temperatures compared with naïve mice following each challenge. Mean temperatures of those mice that had been treated were essentially the same as in naïve mice and significantly higher than in sham-treated mice at each of 7 challenges following the first course, and at the challenge after the second course of treatment. Plasma histamine levels after the second course of treatment were also indistinguishable from those of naïve mice following the final challenge.

Treated mice had persistently lower levels of peanut-specific IgE through week 65. Conversely, peanut-specific IgG2a [IgG (ood)]-blocking antibody levels were significantly increased following 4 weeks of B-FAHF-2 treatment and remained significantly elevated through week 65.

It appeared, therefore, that B-FAHF-2 treatment also suppressed antigen-specific Th2 cytokine secretion and increased Th1 cytokine INF-γ secretion.

When cytokines were assayed, this was borne out. Consistent with the earlier experiments, B-FAHF-2 was shown to modulate B-cell activity in the right direction—up for tolerance-related cytokines, and down for allergenic ones. More studies provided direct evidence that, in vitro, B-FAHF-2 directly suppressed peanut-primed Th2-cell, B-cell and mast-cell activities, suggesting that many mechanisms underlie B-FAHF-2's clinical effects, although the precise

此,小鼠得到了大约12个月的显著保护,这是它们寿命的一半。目前熟悉的临床措施以及观察到的过敏反应迹象均显示出抗过敏作用。在每次刺激后,花生过敏假治疗组小鼠体温都明显低于未处理小鼠。在第一疗程的所有7次刺激后,以及第二疗程后的刺激后,治疗组小鼠的平均体温与未处理组小鼠基本一致,且显著高于假治疗组小鼠。第二个疗程治疗后的血浆组胺水平也与最后一次刺激后未处理组小鼠没有明显区别。

在第65周,治疗组小鼠的花生特异性IgE持续保持在低水平。相反,在B-FAHF-2治疗四周后,花生特异性IgG2a[IgG(好)]抑制的抗体水平显著增加,并且在65周内保持显著上升趋势。

所以,B-FAHF-2治疗似乎抑制了抗原特异性Th2细胞因子的分泌并增加了Th1细胞因子INF-γ的分泌。

当测定细胞因子时,这一点得到了证实。与早期的实验一样,显示B-FAHF-2朝正确方向调节B细胞活性,即对于耐受相关的细胞因子,上调B细胞活性;对于过敏相关的细胞因子,下调B细胞活性。许多研究直接证明,体外B-FAHF-2直接抑制花生致敏的Th2细胞、B细胞和肥大细胞的活性,表明B-FAHF-2的临床疗效隐匿有多种机制,然而,精

mechanisms remain to be determined.

No Sickness, No Death

To test B-FAHF-2 for safety apart from the therapeutic effects, mice were fed 12 times the daily dose and observed for 24 hours. None died or even got sick. Moreover, in the 2 weeks following, there were no signs of altered physical appearance or activity. Blood cell counts and serum liver/kidney function test results were all within the normal range 2 weeks after feeding. Examined under a microscope, tissue samples from the heart, lung, liver, kidney, stomach, and spleen from B-FAHF-2 mice showed nothing unusual. The B-FAHF-2-fed mice were continuously observed over a 65-week period, and none showed signs of altered physical appearance or activity.

Butanol proved so effective at extracting the useful compounds from a complex herbal formula that it points the way for tolerable treatment of food allergies. B-FAHF-2 reduced the effective daily dose for peanut-allergic mice by 80% compared to the water extract (FAHF-2) while retaining excellent efficacy and safety. The therapeutic effect is long-lasting, didn't generate resistance, and acted on multiple cells involved in the allergic response.

Additional in vitro research showed that B-FAHF-2 directly suppressed IgE production by a human B-cell line and activation of rat basophil leukemia (RBL) cells in dosages far below those of FAHF-2. The IC50 (dose that causes 50% inhibition) of B-FAHF-2 was 7.5-fold lower for B-FAHF-2 than for FAHF-2. No cytotoxicity (cell damage) was observed. Because B-FAHF-2 is markedly more convenient for clinical use

确的机制仍有待测定。

试验小鼠没有出现疾病或死亡

除疗效之外,为了检测 B-FAHF-2 的安全性,给小鼠每天喂食 12 倍的日剂量,进行 24 小时观察。没有小鼠死亡甚至患病。而且在接下来的两周内,它们的外表和身体活动未发生任何变化。这样喂食小鼠两周后,检查结果显示血细胞计数和血清肝/肾功能均在正常范围内。在显微镜下观察用 B-FAHF-2 喂食小鼠的心、肺、肝、肾、胃和脾的组织样本,显示无异常情况。连续观察喂食 B-FAHF-2 小鼠超过 65 周,没有显示出外表和身体活动改变的迹象。

事实证明,丁醇在从复杂的中药方剂中提取有用的化合物时非常有效,它为耐受性良好的食物过敏治疗指明了方向。与水提取物(FAHF-2)相比,B-FAHF-2 使花生过敏小鼠的有效日剂量减少了 80%,同时保持了良好的疗效和安全性。治疗效果持久,且不产生耐药性,作用于参与过敏反应的多个细胞。

另一项体外研究发现,采用远低于 FAHF-2 剂量的 B-FAHF-2,通过人体 B 细胞株和大鼠嗜碱性粒细胞白血病(RBL)细胞的活化作用,直接抑制 IgE 的产生。B-FAHF-2 的 IC50(引起 50% 抑制作用的剂量)比 FAHF-2 低 7.5 倍,且未造成细胞毒性(细胞损伤)。因为 B-FAHF-2 在

than is FAHF-2, the team has proposed combining B-FAHF-2 and peanut OIT, with the goal of increasing safety and efficacy of that approach. Food allergy is a complicated epidemic. Meeting the needs of a broad variety of patients will require a portfolio of treatments.

⑮ Documenting the Quest for a Cure

Many mice die as a consequence of laboratory science. So do many trees, because of the reams of paperwork, although I suppose it might be more accurate to say these days that mounds of coal must be burned to crunch all the numbers and record the data electronically.

Any IND—FAHF-2 is known as IND 77468—must be documented in the form of an annual report, which describes the progress that has been made to date and new studies that are being planned. For someone like me, who has only a lay appreciation of the details of such research, the IND annual report provides a useful summary of the knowledge acquired in dozens of peer-reviewed papers. Step-by-step increments are drawn together and condensed.

The October 2012 annual report for the phase-2 trial recounts screening 106 patients at 3 sites, which yielded 68 subjects—a scientific term meaning people.

Again, "first do no harm" is the paramount consideration. The most important data concerns adverse effects. Adverse effects are recorded as "definitely related," "probably related," "possibly

临床上明显比 FAHF-2 方便使用,所以研究小组提出联合 B-FAHF-2 和花生 OIT,目的是增加该方法的安全性和有效性。食物过敏是一种复杂的流行病。满足各种患者的需求将需要一系列的治疗方案。

⑮ 记录对治愈方法的探索

任何科学研究都要付出代价,许多小鼠因为实验室科学而死亡。许多树木因为大量的文书工作而被砍。尽管我认为现在更准确的说法应该是,大量的煤炭被消耗才能产生电能、压缩所有的数据并以电子方式记录数据。

任何试验性新药必须以年度报告形式进行记录、描述已取得进展以及正在规划的新研究项目,而 FAHF-2 被称为试验性新药 77,468。对于像我一样对这种研究的详细资料理解肤浅的外行人,几十篇同行评审论文中得来的有用知识总结,逐步的进展被收集、压缩到试验性新药年度报告。

2012 年 10 月第 2 阶段试验的年度报告叙述了从 3 个地区筛选出 106 例患者,最终得到 68 例受试者("受试者"是一个科学术语,指的是参加试验的人)。

再强调一次,"无损于病人为先"是最重要的事情。最重要的数据涉及一些不良反应。不良反应被记录为"明确相关的""非常可能相关的"

related," and "unrelated."①

The data point that Dr. Li is most proud of is that not a single adverse effect was deemed definitely related to the formula under study. Of the most common symptom (gastrointestinal) 81 were reported, including vomiting, diarrhea, and abdominal pain; only 8 were deemed probably related to the medication, 41 possibly related, and 32 *unrelated*. Of the second most common symptoms (respiratory), only one was deemed possibly related and 74 were *un*related.

Each symptom was investigated by personal physicians as well as by participating doctors. In all, 10 subjects withdrew, 4 of them because of time constraints and difficulty with compliance, and 4 more because of recurrent abdominal pain.

Another prominent item in the annual report was something that had been mentioned in the peer-reviewed studies but that, in this more concise format, loomed larger. Though the various iterations of FAHF up-regulated the production of nonallergenic Th1

"可能相关的"以及"不相关的"。

李秀敏博士最引以为傲的数据是,没有一种不良反应被认为与正在研究的配方明确相关。最常见的症状(胃肠道)81例,包括呕吐、腹泻和腹痛;只有8例非常可能与药物有关,41例可能与药物有关,32例与药物无关。在第二常见的症状(呼吸系统)中,只有一种被认为可能是相关的,74例是不相关的。

私人医生和参与试验的医生研究了各种症状。共10位受试者退出,其中4例因为时间限制和难以实现依从性,4例因为复发的腹痛而退出。

年度报告中的另一个突出点是同行评议研究中所提到的内容,但是在这种更简洁的格式中,显得更重要。尽管FAHF的不同迭代不断上调非过敏反应Th1细胞因子的产生

---

① a. Definitely related: An AE that follows a temporal sequence from administration of the test product and/or procedure; follows a known response pattern to the test article and/or procedure; and, when appropriate to the protocol, is confirmed by improvement after stopping the test product and cannot be reasonably explained by known characteristics of the subject's clinical state or by other therapies.

b. Probably related: An AE that follows a reasonable temporal sequence from administration of the test product and/or procedure; follows a known response pattern to the test product and/or procedure; and cannot be reasonably explained by the known characteristics of the participant's clinical state or other therapies.

c. Possibly related: An AE that follows a reasonable temporal sequence from administration of the test product and/or procedure and follows a known response pattern to the test product and/or procedure, but could have been produced by the participant's clinical state or by other therapies.

Not associated: An AE for which sufficient information exists to indicate that the etiology is not related to the test product and/or therapy.

d. Unrelated: An AE that does not follow a reasonable temporal sequence after administration of the test product and/or procedure and most likely is explained by the participant's clinical disease state or by other therapies. (IND 77468 Phase 1 for B-FAHF-2)

cytokines and down-regulated those of Th2, they accomplished this with no cytotoxicity to the PBMCs. That is, there was no "collateral damage" to cells that might play a critical role in maintaining a strong immune system. This adds to the appeal of herbal medicines' ability to restore balance to the bodies of mice and people without damaging anything important, as opposed to, say, antibiotics, which we now know destroy good bacteria as well as harmful ones, something associated in theory with one aspect of the rise of the allergy epidemic.

Refining FAHF-2 Allows Researchers to Isolate and Understand Effectiveness of Active Compounds

Using butanol to refine FAHF-2 not only makes it possible to reduce the daily dosage from 30 pills to 6—a must for eventual clinical use—but also makes possible characterization and purification of the active compounds. This allows us to understand which of the ingredients are doing what.

The annual report documents this activity in great detail: Isolation of 4 fractional compounds from B-FAHF-2 based on their polarity using a "preparative HPLC system" showed that the different compounds contributed to inhibiting the allergic response in different ways. The "alkaloid-rich fraction 2 (F2) inhibited IgE production and mast-cell degranulation *in vitro*" while fractions 3 and 4 (F3, F4), rich in *flavonoids* and *triterpenes*, inhibited TNF-α production, which contributes to inflammation. Two compounds from F2 demonstrated that "*berberine* is the most potent active compound in F2 that inhibits IgE production, mast-cell degranulation, and Th2 cytokine production." Using HPLC to create chemical

以及下调 Th2 的产生,同时未对外周血单核细胞造成细胞毒性。也就是,对可能在维持较强免疫系统中发挥重要作用的细胞不会产生"附带损害"。这增加了中草药的吸引力,因为它能恢复小鼠或人的身体平衡能力,而又不会损伤任何重要功能。相反,抗生素,我们都知道它既破坏有益菌,也破坏有害菌,在理论上它与过敏流行病上升的某方面有关。

提纯 FAHF-2 让研究人员分离并理解活性化合物的有效性

采用丁醇精炼 FAHF-2,不仅有可能将日剂量从 30 粒降低至 6 粒——对于最终临床应用是必须的,还有可能表征和提纯活性化合物。这让我们了解各个成分所起的作用。

年度报告中详细记录了这一活性:根据化合物的极性,采用"制备型高效液相色谱系统",将 4 种分馏化合物从 B-FAHF-2 中分离出来,结果显示不同化合物通过不同方式抑制过敏反应。"富含生物碱的组分 2 (F2)可以抑制 IgE 的产生和肥大细胞的体外脱粒",而富含黄酮类和三萜类的组分 3 和 4(F3 和 F4),可以抑制导致炎症的 TNF-α 的产生。来自 F2 的两种化合物表明,"黄连素是 F2 中最有效的活性化合物,它可以抑制 IgE 的产生、肥大细胞的脱粒以及 Th2 细胞因子的产生"。采用

"fingerprints," the peaks of F3 and F4 were found to correspond to those of *Ling Zhi* (*Ganoderma Luciderm*), the magic mushroom. So far, 15 compounds have been isolated and characterized from *Ling Zhi* itself. We are a long way from the story of the white snake.

B-FAHF-2 was also analyzed for heavy metals, pesticides, and microbes and was found to fall within acceptable limits. In addition, the placebo tablets had to meet safety standards.

Thus, the stage was set for a new trial within precise parameters: 18 patients randomized to receive 4 tablets of B-FAHF-2 bid (twice a day) for 7 days, double-blind. Corn-flour placebo tablets are produced by the same manufacturer that produced the B-FAHF-2 active drug.

The report describes the procedure in great detail: "The initial evaluation will consist of a thorough medical history and physical examination; vital signs— blood pressure, heart and breathing rate, body temperature; prick-skin testing to peanut, individual tree nuts, sesame and/or individual fish or shellfish; total IgE level; peanut-specific, tree nut-specific, sesame-specific, and/or fish- or shellfish-specific IgE level; baseline spirometry; electrocardiogram; urinalysis; and pregnancy test and routine laboratory blood tests (complete blood count, serum chemistries, renal function, liver function tests). Subjects will be instructed to complete a symptom diary while they are participating in the trial. The clinical site investigators will be in direct telephone contact with each subject

高效液相色谱构建化学"指纹图谱",发现 F3 和 F4 的峰值与神奇蘑菇灵芝的峰值一致。到目前为止,已经分离出 15 种具有灵芝特征的化合物。《白蛇传》中描述灵芝具有起死回生的作用,但要揭示其中的机制,我们还需要做很多工作。

同时对 B-FAHF-2 进行了重金属、农药和微生物分析,发现其含量在可接受范围内。另外,安慰剂药片必须满足安全标准。

因此,精确参数下的新试验已经准备好了:18 例患者随机服用 4 片 B-FAHF-2(每日两次),共 7 天,双盲。玉米粉安慰剂药片和 B-FAHF-2 活性药品来自同一个生产厂家。

报告详细描述了试验流程:"初步评估包括:详尽的病史和体检;生命体征包括血压、心率和呼吸频率、体温;采用花生、个别坚果、芝麻和/或个别鱼类或贝类进行的皮肤点刺试验;IgE 总水平;花生特异性、坚果特异性、芝麻特异性和/或鱼类或贝类特异性的 IgE 水平;基准肺活量测定;心电图;尿液分析;以及妊娠测试和实验室血常规检查(全血细胞计数、血清生化检验、肾功能、肝功能检查)。参与试验时,受试者将在指导下填写症状日志。临床现场的调查员大约每隔一天,就会直接电话联系每一位受试者。同时,一名研究内科

approximately every other day. Also, a study physician will be on call to discuss possible AEs by telephone. During the final visit of the acute phase-1 trial, the investigators will review the larger status of subject health, including the symptom diary. The final visit will incorporate a physical examination, vital signs, spirometry, electrocardiogram, urinalysis, and routine laboratory blood tests (complete blood count, serum chemistries, renal function, liver function tests)."

Prior to the start of the acute phase-1 trial, aliquots of peripheral blood mononuclear cells will be treated in vitro with B-FAHF-2 to determine the direct effect of B-FAHF-2 or its compounds on T-cell cytokine profiles and histamine release by basophils. Furthermore, B-FAHF-2 effects on cytokine and transcription factor gene expression and regulation including epigenetic regulation of T cells will be determined.

The FDA has now given approval for using B-FAHF-2 to replace FAHF-2 for the clinical study. A new acute phase-1 study will be initiated, but because FAHF-2 showed excellent safety data, the team doesn't have to go back to square one to establish safety. The dose will be 8 tablets daily to ease clinical administration and compliance and to allow a longer duration of treatment that is more comparable to the murine experiments. (Note: Documentation is being prepared as of this writing)

医生随时待命准备通过电话讨论可能的不良事件。在急性第1阶段试验的最后一次回访中,调查员会审查关于受试者健康的更多项目,包括症状日志。最后一次回访包含体检、生命体征、肺活量测定、心电图、尿液分析和实验室血常规检查(全血细胞计数、血清生化检验、肾功能和肝功能检查)。"

在急性第1阶段试验开始之前,先将等分的几份外周血单核细胞进行 B-FAHF-2 体外处理,然后测定 B-FAHF-2 或其化合物对 T 细胞因子谱和嗜碱性粒细胞释放的组胺的直接影响。此外,还将测定 B-FAHF-2 对细胞因子和转录因子的基因表达和调节,包括 T 细胞的表观遗传调控的影响。

目前,FDA 已经批准可以使用 B-FAHF-2 取代 FAHF-2 进行临床研究。新的急性第1阶段试验即将开始,但是因为 FAHF-2 显示极好的安全数据,所以研究小组不需要从头开始去确定其安全性。日剂量将降低至 8 粒,有利于临床给药和依从性,并且允许有更长的持续治疗时间,更可与小鼠实验相媲美。(注:截至写作本书时,证明文件正在准备中)

PART THREE

The Future

As we await the results of the latest phase of FAHF-2 trials, it's not too early to peer into the future and think about other dimensions suggested by Dr. Li's work. Each of the final five chapters focuses on a different element of the ongoing story, from very practical extensions of the research just described to breathtaking concepts suggested by new insights into the nature of the immune system.

Multiple Food Allergies for the Price of One

OIT may prove practical for a certain proportion of food-allergic patients—probably those who are allergic to a single allergen and have no problems with eosinophils in their digestive tracts—but what of those who have many food allergies? Quite apart from the difficulties of assessing the progress for any individual allergen, there's the problem of continually subjecting these patients to known irritants. The alternative is to modulate the immune system itself.

From One Generation to the Next

Many parents wonder how life-threatening allergies can emerge mysteriously in very small children. Although a genetic predisposition to allergies is accepted science, the new science of epigenetics is starting to reveal how the environment, diet, and behavior can affect the way our genes are expressed and that these subtle alterations can be passed to

第三部分

前　景

当我们等待 FAHF-2 试验最新阶段的结果时,现在展望未来并考虑李秀敏博士的工作所建议的其他方面已经不算太早。在最后五个章节中,每一篇都聚焦于正在进行研究的不同方面,从所述研究的实际延伸到对免疫系统本质的新洞察力所提出的令人惊叹的概念。

一药多治

OIT 可能得到证实对一定比例的食物过敏患者很实用,可能这些患者对单一过敏原过敏,并且他们消化道内的嗜酸性细胞并没有出现异常情况。然而,那些对多种食物过敏的患者怎么办呢? 除了很难对各个过敏原进行评估,还有一个问题就是要让患者不断地接触已知刺激物。另一种选择是调节免疫系统本身。

从一代遗传到下一代

许多父母想知道,威胁生命的过敏症状是如何莫名其妙地发生在很小的孩子身上。尽管过敏的遗传易感性是公认的科学,但是表观遗传学这一新兴科学开始揭示环境、饮食和行为如何能够影响基因表达,以及这些微妙的变化如何传递给下一代。

offspring. This chapter not only documents how detrimental changes can be passed on but also shows that it may be possible to reverse such transmission in the future.

本篇不仅纪实性地描述了有害的变化如何传递给下一代,而且显示在将来有可能会逆转这种传播。

Beyond Food Allergies

One of the most exciting things about the East-meets-West paradigm is that we not only can see that these herbal compounds work but can also determine why they work. Instead of measuring the effect of a single molecule on a single molecule or a single pathway, we can see how a complex compound works on multiple compounds and pathways that are part of other pathologies. This chapter looks at the way Dr. Li's research is finding currency outside the strict realm of allergies.

应用于食物过敏之外的疾病的可能

关于中西医结合的范例,最令人激动的一件事就是我们不仅能够看到这些草药混合物起作用,而且能够确定它们为什么有这些作用。我们没有测定单一分子对单一分子或单一路径的作用,而是能够看见复杂化合物如何影响作为其他病理一部分的多种化合物和多条路径。本篇着眼于李秀敏博士的研究发现应用于过敏疾病之外的其他疾病的前景。

Treating Severe Allergic Diseases: Three Cases from Private Clinical Practice

As Dr. Scott Sicherer tells his colleagues, in China, TCM is just medicine. In her private clinic, Dr. Li regularly uses medicines that are approved as supplements to treat severe allergic diseases apparently with great success. This chapter gives anecdotal accounts of three successful treatments of debilitating and life-threatening allergic cases that have restored joy to the lives of young patients.

治疗严重的过敏疾病:李秀敏私人诊所的三个案例

正如斯科特·史可瑞博士告诉他的同事说,中医在中国就是医学。李秀敏博士在自己的私人诊所,定期使用已批准为补充剂的药物来治疗严重的过敏疾病,并取得了显著成功。本章列举了3个治疗成功的过敏性病例,这些案例中的年轻患者从虚弱无比、生命处于威胁到重拾生活的快乐。

The Slow Road to Clinical Practice

This final chapter grapples with the shortcomings of traditional allergy treatment and research and outlines a possible roadmap for accelerating the practice of integrative medicine—the adoption of TCM-based drugs by a wider population of traditional allergists.

缓慢的临床实践之路

最后一篇努力克服传统过敏治疗和研究的不足之处,并且勾勒出加速整合医学实践的可能路线图,即更多传统的过敏症专科医生采用以中药为基础的药物。

⑫ Multiple Food Allergies for the Price of One

Although peanut allergy gets most of the attention, there remain seven other *major* food allergens—dairy, tree nuts, eggs, shellfish, fish, soy, wheat—and dozens more minor ones. Any of these has the capacity to provoke anaphylaxis—that is, a combination of symptoms in more than one organ system (skin, respiratory, digestive), which can be life- threatening. Most research into desensitization against food allergies has concentrated on one allergen at a time. Unlike immunotherapy for environmental allergies, for which multiple allergens can be injected together, experiments with OIT for food allergies have concentrated on single allergens because of the different profiles of the different foods. Approximately 20% of children outgrow their peanut, shellfish, fish, and tree-nut allergies, whereas 80% outgrow their milk and egg allergies. ① Studies are inconclusive for milk allergies in particular as to whether OIT is responsible for desensitization or whether it has taken place on its own since 80% outgrow them. ②

Then, too, the proteins in different foods may be altered by cooking, sometimes making them less allergenic, or sometimes more. Ara h2, which is one of the big-three peanut allergens, seems to be strengthened by roasting (the dominant method of preparation in the United States) and weakened by boiling, frying, and pickling, which are more common in Korea. Ara h1 and Ara h3, however, are not affected, so this doesn't

⑫ 一药多治

尽管花生过敏受到了很多关注，但还有另外 7 种主要的食物过敏原包括奶制品、坚果、蛋类、贝类、鱼类、大豆和小麦——以及其他几十种次要食物过敏原。任何一种都能够引起过敏反应，即在多种器官系统（皮肤、呼吸系统和消化系统）中的能够威胁生命的系列症状。大多数对食物过敏的脱敏研究每次仅专注于一种过敏原。不像针对环境过敏的免疫疗法那样可以同时注射多种过敏原，采用 OIT 治疗食物过敏的实验专注于单一过敏原，因为不同食物具有不同的结构。大约 20% 的儿童长大后不再对花生、贝类、鱼类和坚果过敏，而 80% 的儿童长大后不再对牛奶和蛋类过敏。对于牛奶过敏的研究尚无定论，尤其关于 OIT 是否是脱敏的原因还是患者长大后自行发生脱敏，毕竟有 80% 儿童长大后脱敏。

此外，烹饪可能会使不同食物中的蛋白质发生变化，有时会减弱或加强它们的致敏性。Ara h2 是三种主要花生过敏原中的一种，烘焙（美国的主要烹饪方法）似乎会加强其致敏性，而在韩国比较常见的煮、炸和腌制可以减弱其致敏性。Ara h1 和 Ara h3 不受影响，所以烹饪方法产生不了太多保护。这些成分与致敏性

---

① NIAID-Sponsored Expert Panel. Guidelines for the diagnosis and management of food allergy in the United States: report of the NIAID-Sponsored Expert Panel[J]. The Journal of Allergy and Clinical Immunology, 2010, 126(6): S1 - S58.

② Brozek J L, Terracciano L, Hsu J, et al. Oral immunotherapy for IgE-mediated cow's milk allergy: a systematic review and meta-analysis [J]. Clinical & Experimental Allergy, 2012 (3): 363 - 374. See more at http://www. asthmaallergieschildren. com/2012/05/ll/oral- immunotherapy-for-food-allergy-not-ready-for-prime- time/# sthash. CeusCFfJ. dpuf.

constitute much protection.① The important variable between these components and the less-allergenic Ara h6 and Ara h8 is that the more dangerous proteins are harder to digest and are more likely to survive intact and be absorbed, allowing them to circulate and cause systemic reaction. For kids with peanut allergies, no method of cooking changes the proteins sufficiently, but baking eggs or milk may help the child allergic to these foods.

Between the different molecular profiles of various allergens, the tendency for patients to outgrow at different rates, and so on, assembling a homogeneous sample for a single food study is hard enough. For multiple allergens, it would be far more difficult.

One answer is to attack the problem from the other direction—the production of antibodies without regard for specific allergies. All these allergies have something in common: the Th2-IgE mediated response. The most promising line of OIT for multiple food allergies uses omalizumab to speed the process of desensitization. This research is being conducted under the direction of Dr. Kari Nadeau of Stanford.

Omalizumab works by binding a particular epitope on the handle-like portion of IgE antibodies so they can no longer attach to their allergen-specific high-affinity receptors on the mast cell. They become, in effect, square pegs that can no longer fit in their round holes. This gives IgG(ood)4 blocking antibodies the chance to occupy these receptors without competition from IgE (vil). Because all IgE antibodies have the same handle, it should work with all of them. Thus, the doctor can theoretically supply all the allergens at

小的 Ara h6 和 Ara h8 之间的重要变量是,更危险的蛋白质更难消化,并且更有可能原封不动地存活并被吸收,进而得以在体内循环而引起全身反应。对于花生过敏患儿而言,没有任何烹饪方式可以充分地改变蛋白质,但是烘焙鸡蛋或牛奶可能会引发他们对这些食物产生过敏反应。

由于不同过敏原具有不同的分子结构,以及患儿在成长时克服过敏的概率也不同,很难为单一食物过敏研究收集同一种样本。对于多种过敏而言就更难了。

一种办法是从另一个方向着手,即不考虑特异性过敏原而考虑抗体的产生。所有这些过敏原具有一个共同的特点:均是 Th2-IgE 介导的反应。治疗多种食物过敏的 OIT 最值得期待的方法是采用奥马珠单抗加速脱敏过程。该研究在斯坦福大学的卡利·纳多博士指导下进行。

奥马珠单抗的工作原理是将特定的表位结合在 IgE 抗体的手柄状部分上,因此,它们不能附着在肥大细胞上的过敏特异性高亲和力受体上。这就好像,它们变成方形的钉子,不能再装进圆孔里了。这使(好)IgG4 阻断抗体有机会在不与(坏)IgE 竞争的情况下占据这些受体。因为所有 IgE 抗体都具有同样的手柄,所以奥马珠单抗应该对所有 IgE 都有效。因此,理论上,医生能够同时提供所有过敏原,并且所有

---

① Lee, et al. , op cit.

once, and all the IgE will be rendered harmless long enough for the IgG4 blocking antibodies to occupy all the receptors. This universal effect has led to omalizumab being studied for off-label treatment of other allergic conditions besides asthma, particularly chronic urticaria—really bad recurring hives.

Promising though this combination therapy sounds, omalizumab has a few drawbacks, as mentioned earlier. One is that it is itself a protein to which a few people can become allergic. Another is cost, approximately $ 1,000 per month, possibly forever, which makes it economical to use mainly for severe asthmatics who would otherwise be hospitalized frequently, costing their insurance companies much more. A third drawback is that omalizumab may not improve on the likely weakness of OIT in general—namely, that it only wears out current Th2 cells but its effects may be temporary. Although OIT does inhibit basophil activity for a period,[①] which helps reduce reactivity, the major food allergies often last a lifetime, even without any exposure. Once desensitization is achieved, it may be possible to maintain it with doses of the offending food only, not the $ 1000 drug. Annoying though it may be to take daily doses of single foods to maintain desensitization, having to incorporate peanuts, egg, wheat, and shrimp into one's everyday diet, to name just one combination, will require considerable culinary ingenuity, however.

IgE 都会在足够长的时间内变得无害,以便 IgG4 阻断抗体能占据所有的受体。这一普遍作用已经导致了奥马珠单抗被用于除哮喘之外的其他过敏疾病的标签外治疗(标签外使用是指将药物用于未经批准的适应证或在未经批准的年龄组、剂量或给药方式下使用药物。)的研究,尤其是慢性荨麻疹,那种严重的复发性荨麻疹的研究。

尽管这种结合疗法听起来很有希望,但如前所述,奥马珠单抗仍有一些弊端。一是它本身是一种让少数人产生过敏反应的蛋白质。二是它的成本,可能需要每月大约 1000 美元,而且是永久性的。这主要对严重哮喘患者比较经济实惠,否则住院治疗将使他们的保险公司报销更多费用。三是奥马珠单抗可能不会改进 OIT 的弱点,即它会耗尽现有的 Th2 细胞,但是它的效果可能是暂时的。尽管 OIT 会抑制嗜碱性粒细胞活性一段时间,但这有利于降低反应度,但即使不接触过敏原,主要的食物过敏也经常会持续一生。但是一旦实现脱敏,就有可能只用过敏原食物的剂量,而不是 1000 美元的药物。但是将不同食材纳入日常饮食本身就需要相当多的烹饪技巧,比如花生、鸡蛋、小麦和虾的组合。

---

① Jones S M, Pons L, Roberts J L, et al. Clinical efficacy and immune regulation with peanut oral immunotherapy[J]. Journal of Allergy and Clinical Immunology, 2009, 124(2): 292 – 300.

A newer foray into combination therapy is the brainchild of Dr. Nadeau and Dr. Li, using FAHF-2 as the adjunct in the place of omalizumab. I had the privilege of sitting at lunch with the two of them and watching them outline the study on the back of a napkin. [1] It must be said that the science of food allergies is too new and patient phenotypes are too varied to concentrate all the funding and scientific talent too early in the process. It is very likely that food-allergy patients will be varied enough so that treatment will entail a range of methods. (Note： another therapy called Viaskin®, or the " peanut patch", in which measured doses of peanut extract are applied to the skin, is in trials at various medical centers, including Mount Sinai.)

The sole trial of a single therapy for multiple food allergies is being conducted by Dr. Li and colleagues at Mount Sinai and in Dallas at the University of Texas Southwestern Medical Center and Children's Medical Center. They began a new subproject of their phase-1 trial[2] to test butanol-refined FAHF-2 with subjects aged 6 to 45 who are allergic to one or more foods including peanut, tree nut, sesame, fish, or shellfish as documented by a positive skin test and/or food allergen-specific IgE level for the allergens. ［The protocol for the experiment reads：" The initial evaluation will consist of a thorough medical history and physical examination；vital signs；prick skin testing to peanut, individual tree nuts, sesame, and/or

纳多博士和李秀敏博士尝试了一次新的联合疗法,采用 FAHF-2 来辅助奥马珠单抗。我非常荣幸与他们两位共进午餐,看他们用浅显的语言为我这个外行人介绍了这个研究的情况。不得不说食物过敏学科太新颖,患者类型变化多端,所以不太可能在这个领域投入很多经费和科学人员。而且食物过敏患者很可能会出现各种不同情况,以至于治疗必须包括很多方法。(注:另一种疗法称为 Viaskin® 或"花生修补",此法是将一定剂量的花生提取物涂在皮肤上,这种方法正在各个医疗中心包括西奈山医院中进行试验。)

李秀敏博士和其同事在西奈山医院和位于达拉斯的得克萨斯大学西南医学中心和儿童医学中心,正进行治疗多种食物过敏的单一疗法的唯一试验。他们开始了第 1 阶段的一个新的子项目,采用丁醇提纯的 FAHF-2 治疗过敏患者(6 ~ 45 岁)。这些患者对一种或多种食物过敏,包括花生、坚果、芝麻、鱼类或贝类,这些都由皮试结果呈阳性以及/或食物过敏特异性 IgE 水平证明。[实验方案记录:"初步评估将包括详尽的病史和体检;生命体征;采用花生、单个

---

① http://www.asthmaallergieschildren.com/2013/04/20/history-is-made-at-lunch/.

② IND 77468 Phase 1 for B-FAHF-2.

individual fish or shellfish; total IgE level; peanut-specific, tree nut-specific, sesame-specific, and/or fish- or shellfish-specific IgE level; baseline spirometry; electrocardiogram; urinalysis; pregnancy test and routine laboratory blood tests (complete blood count, serum chemistries, renal function, liver function tests)."] Individuals with a history of anaphylaxis to these allergens were excluded (the object of the trial being not to cure the subjects but to examine the underlying functioning of the immune system) along with many other immune disorders and other medical conditions. Subjects will keep symptom diaries in addition to being in regular touch with study personnel.

Opening up this test to a spectrum of allergies also makes it easier to recruit subjects who meet the desired parameters. This is, in a way, the inverse of the murine model of testing. With mice, it made sense to induce allergies to a lone allergen, instead of several, and to treat them with single drug.

If this test succeeds, it will assess several things. First, it will further establish the safety of B-FAHF-2. Second, it will show that the up-regulation of Th1 cytokines and production of IgG antibodies and inhibition of Th2-IgE was general, not specific to peanuts.

⓭ From One Generation to the Next
▌ "What did I do wrong?"

Many mothers of food-allergic children ask themselves that question continually from the time of diagnosis. Although the tendency of allergies to run in families is long established, the onset of life-threatening

坚果、芝麻和/或个别鱼类或贝类进行皮肤点刺试验;IgE 总水平;花生特异、坚果特异、芝麻特异和/或鱼类或贝类特异的 IgE 水平;基准肺活量测定;心电图;尿液分析;妊娠试验和实验室血常规检查(全血细胞计数、血清生化检验、肾功能和肝功能检查)。"]对这些过敏原有过敏史的患者被剔除(试验目的不是治愈受试者,而是检查免疫系统的潜在功能,并伴随许多其他免疫紊乱和其他医疗状况)。除与研究人员保持定期联系外,受试者还将填写症状日记。

将这个测试扩展到多种过敏的范围也使招募符合所需参数的受试者变得更容易。在某种程度上,这与小鼠模型的测试相反。对小鼠进行单一过敏原的过敏诱导,而不是多种过敏原的过敏诱导,并用单一药物治疗更有意义。

如果试验成功,它将评估几个方面。首先,它将进一步确立 B-FAHF-2 的安全性。其次,它将显示 Th1 细胞因子的上调、IgG 抗体的产生以及 Th2-IgE 的抑制作用是普遍的,不仅仅针对花生。

⓭ 从一代遗传到下一代
▌ "我是不是做错了什么?"

可能在确诊后,许多食物过敏儿童的母亲都会不断问自己这个问题。尽管过敏在家族中代代相传的趋势早已确立,但即使在有环境过敏和哮

food allergies in a new generation is a shock even in families with a history of environmental allergies and asthma. Food allergies become the basis of a blame game. Mothers, fathers, in-laws—no one's genes or neurotic tendencies escape scrutiny. Privately, however, (or in the extended privacy of closed Facebook groups where I meet them), mothers pick over their gestational diets, medications they took or allowed to be given to their children, whether or not they breast-fed, how long they breast-fed; these and many other things must have been their own fault, they believe.

Self-recrimination, however, is not only a recipe for personal misery but is also wide of the mark. There is likely no single maternal behavior that has a one-to-one relationship to a child's allergies. The conventional wisdom on maternal diet—to eat certain foods, especially peanuts, or avoid them—has flip-flopped, and continuing research is equivocal. Other factors such as caesarian delivery and use of antibiotics indicate that with disruption of the natural microbe environment in a newborn, the immune system is disturbed along with it, but until now, who was to know? And let's give the moms a break. What choice did they have? These were mostly lifesaving interventions, although many caesarians have been performed for "convenience." Attempts to restore a measure of balance through supplements such as probiotics and vitamins are not yet at the point where there is any clear road to correction.

Allergies do appear to get worse in succeeding generations：sneezing leads to wheezing, which leads to anaphylaxis. As mentioned in chapter 1, Dr. Susan Prescott has written that the allergy epidemic is likely

喘病史的家庭中，新一代威胁生命的食物过敏的发作依然令他们震惊。食物过敏会让家庭成员互相责备。母亲、父亲、姻亲们——他们的基因或神经过敏趋势都不会逃过审查。但是，私下地，（或者在我遇见她们的Facebook封闭群组中，在更大的隐私范围内），母亲们选择妊娠期饮食、选择她们服用的药物或允许给孩子服用的药物，不论她们是否喂食母乳、喂食多长时间；她们认为，这些事情和其他许多事情都是她们的过错。

然而，自我谴责不仅会造成个人痛苦，还是离谱的。因为母亲的任何一个行为与孩子的过敏可能都没有一一对应的关系。关于母亲饮食的传统观念（食用某些食物，尤其是花生，或避免食用）已经发生了翻天覆地的改变，继续进行的研究结果不明。剖宫产和使用抗生素等因素表明，随着新生儿体内的自然微生物环境的破坏，免疫系统也随之受到干扰，但是直到现在，谁知道答案呢？让我们给母亲们一个喘息的时间。她们有什么选择？尽管大部分剖宫产是为了"方便"，但这些干预措施主要是拯救生命。通过补充益生菌和维生素等恢复平衡的尝试，当下还不能算作有效的途径。

在后代中出现的过敏症会更严重：打喷嚏会导致喘息，进而导致过敏。如第1篇所述，苏珊·普莱斯考特博士已经写到，过敏性疾病可能是

the product of multiple assaults on our skin, sinuses, lungs, and digestive systems—anywhere our immune systems confront the environment. Furthermore, these assaults may accumulate from one generation to the next as toxins affect gene expression—not the genes themselves—a process called epigenetics, or "above the genome." Chris Faulk, a postdoctoral fellow studying environmental epigenetics and evolution, writes in an online article: "We know that environmental changes by toxicant exposure, stress, nutrition, and other factors can alter the epigenetic marks of many body tissues, including the gametes, and so an intergenerational epigenetic effect can be seen."[1] Thus, a child's asthma may be attributable in part to the mother's life in a city with high levels of "black carbon" from diesel fumes[2] or to a grandmother's smoking habit.[3] Families with no recorded history of allergies may become allergic, and mild allergies can get worse. My own surmise is that if humans can share 99% of our genome with mice, we can also share genetic tendencies with other human beings and that a family history with no known tendency to allergies is just a few gene expressions away from one that does have allergies. This is not the same as Lamarckism, named for Jean-Baptiste Lamarck, "who, beginning in the early 1800s (sic), put forth the hypothesis that giraffes could pass on long necks to their offspring by stretching their own necks throughout their lives..."[4] It is instead the subtle influence of chemicals on the biochemical processes that comprise the immune system.

我们的任何免疫系统面对环境(皮肤、鼻窦、肺和消化系统)受到多次攻击的产物。而且,这些攻击可能从这一代积累到下一代,就像毒素影响基因表达一样,但不是基因本身,这个过程被称为表观遗传学,或"基因组之上"。克里斯·福克是一位研究环境表观遗传学和进化的博士后,他在网上一篇文章中写道:"我们知道,由毒物接触、压力、营养和其他因素导致的环境变化能改变许多身体组织的外基因标记,包括胚胎,所以可以看见代际表观遗传效应。"因此,儿童哮喘可能部分归因于母亲生活在柴油烟雾"黑碳"含量高的城市或祖母的吸烟习惯。没有过敏史的家族可能会变得过敏,轻度过敏可能会加重。我猜测,如果我们和小鼠有99%的相同基因组,那么我们也能与他人有相同的遗传趋势,而没有已知过敏倾向的家族史与确实有过敏的家族史只有几个基因表达的距离。这不同于以让·巴蒂斯特·拉马克命名的拉马克学说,"自19世纪早期开始,他提出一种假设,即,长颈鹿能够通过拉伸自己的脖子而将长脖子遗传给下一代……"这与化学物对包含免疫系统的生物化学过程的微妙影响正好相反。

① http://www.mindthesciencegap.Org/2013/06/21/lamarck-lysenko-and-modern-day-epigenetics/.

② Kari N, Cameron M-H, Elizabeth M N, et al. Ambient air pollution impairs regulatory T-cell function in asthma[J]. Journal of Allergy and Clinical Immunology, 2010, 126(4): 845－852.

③ John S T, Virender K R. An epigenetic "smoking gun" for reproductive inheritance[J]. Expert Review of Obstetrics & Gynecology, 2013, 8(2): 99－101.

④ Faulk, op cit.

The bright side of Prescott's thesis is that the epigenetic cascade that has caused an epidemic of allergies and other noncommunicable inflammatory diseases didn't really start all that long ago and so might be at least partially correctable over a relatively brief time frame as well.

Toward Intergenerational Correction

The possibility of curing food allergies and passing the change on to the next generation was demonstrated in a 2009 study by Dr. Li and her Mount Sinai colleagues.[①] After peanut allergy was induced in female mice by the now-familiar method, they were bred with naïve males. A subset of these mothers received low doses of peanut and adjuvant cholera toxin during pregnancy and lactation.

At the age of 5 weeks, the offspring were challenged intragastrically with peanut extract delivered directly through a tube. This was the first exposure to the peanut allergens, so any reaction at all would indicate that allergy can be inherited, but any difference in the degree of reaction would also indicate that protection could also be inherited.

The results were dramatic: 80% of those offspring whose mothers had not received the low doses of peanuts experienced anaphylaxis, compared to just 24% of those that had. There were corresponding changes in body temperature—lower in the more allergic mice, closer to normal in the less reactive. Concentrations of the "good" blocking antibody IgG2 were greater in the offspring of the mothers that had

普莱斯考特论点的有利方面是引起过敏流行病和其他非传染炎症疾病的表观遗传学中的级联反应并不是很久以前就开始的,所以在相对较短的时间内,至少在一定程度上是可以纠正的。

朝代际纠正努力

李秀敏博士和她的西奈山同事在 2009 年的一项研究中证明了治愈食物过敏并将这种变化传递给下一代的可能性。采用现在熟悉的方法,对雌性小鼠进行花生过敏的诱导,然后让它们与未处理的雄性小鼠繁殖。在雌性小鼠的妊娠期和哺乳期,给其中一些小鼠喂食少量花生和佐剂霍乱毒素。

对 5 周龄幼鼠用导管输送花生提取物以进行胃内刺激。这是其第一次接触花生过敏原,所以任何反应都表明过敏可以遗传,但是不同程度的反应表明抗过敏保护也是可以遗传的。

结果很明显:在未接受低剂量花生诱导的雌性小鼠的幼鼠中,80%出现过敏性反应,而接受花生诱导的雌性小鼠幼鼠中,只有 24% 出现过敏性反应。体温也出现相应变化——严重过敏的小鼠体温低,轻度过敏反应的小鼠体温接近正常值。在喂食花生辅剂的小鼠幼鼠体内的"良好"

① Ivan L-E, Ying S, Kirsi M J, et al. Maternal peanut exposure during pregnancy and Lactation reduces peanut allergy risk in offspring[J]. Journal of Allergy and Clinical Immunology, 2009, 124(5): 1039 − 1049.

been dosed with the peanut-adjuvant dosing. Production of Th2 cytokines associated with peanut allergies was significantly lower in the offspring of treated mothers than in those of naïve mothers. This suggested that the right intervention might also mitigate the transmission of the allergy in humans, although it would be impractical to do the same experiment in prospective mothers.

Was this change the result of what we might call " corrective epigenetics," or could some other phenomenon have been at work, such as milk from lactating mothers? Dr. Li says, "This is an excellent question. We have not fed pups on sham mothers yet, but we looked at the neonatal spleen DNA methylation status and found hyper-methylation (repression) of IL-4 promotion at CpG sites * [1]of pups from mothers fed peanuts and cholera toxin, even before peanut sensitization." A paper recounting this study is being prepared as of this writing.

A 2010 experiment[2] using the herbal asthma drug ASHMI—also developed by Dr. Li and her team—lent additional credence to the idea that the heritability of allergies can be blocked by intervention. ASHMI is an extract of 3 herbs—*Ling Zhi*, *Ku Shen* (*Radix Sophora Flavescentis*), and *Gan Cao* (*Radix Glycyirhiza Uralensis*)—that exhibits a " broad spectrum of

阻断抗体 IgG2 的浓度较高。经治疗的雌性小鼠幼鼠中,与花生过敏有关的 Th2 细胞因子的含量显著低于未处理的雌性小鼠幼鼠中的含量。尽管在准妈妈身上进行同样的试验是不切实际的,但是这个结果可以表明,适当的干预也可能缓解人类过敏症的遗传。

这种改变就是我们所说的"矫正表观遗传学"的结果吗? 或者,其他现象起到作用了吗? 比如哺乳期雌性小鼠的乳汁。李秀敏博士说:"这个问题问得很好,我们没有喂食假治疗组雌性小鼠的幼鼠,但是我们观察了新生小鼠脾脏 DNA 的甲基化状态,发现甚至在花生致敏之前,喂食花生和霍乱毒素小鼠的幼鼠的 CpG 部位 IL-4 促进的超甲基化(抑制)。"在写作本书时,详述本研究的论文正在准备中。

2010 年,一项也是由李博士及其团队开发的采用中药 ASHMI 治疗哮喘的实验,为通过干预可以阻断过敏症的遗传性这一观点提供了额外的证据。ASHMI 是 3 种草药(灵芝、苦参和甘草) 的提取物,它展示

---

① ＊CpG sites are regions of DNA where a cytosine nucleotide occurs next to a guanine nucleotide. This is part of the epigenome, the "clothing" of the DNA, described in chapter 1, whose response to certain stimuli determines gene expression—that is, turns the gene on or off.

　CpG 部位是 DNA 上紧挨着鸟嘌呤核苷酸的胞嘧啶核苷酸。这是表观基因组的一部分,是 DNA 的"衣服"(在第一篇中已描述过) ,这些部位对于特定刺激的回应决定着基因表达——也就是,控制着基因的开合。

② Lopez-Exposito I, Birmingham N, Castillo A, et al. ASHMI (Anti-Asthma Herbal Medicine Intervention) prevents maternal transmission of early onset of allergic airway inflammation and mucus cell development in offspring (abstract) [J]. Journal of Allergy and Clinical Immunology, 2010, 125(2): S120.

therapeutic effects on the major pathogenic mechanisms of asthma—airway hyperreactivity, pulmonary inflammation, and airway remodeling—as well as downregulating Th2 responses and direct modulation of airway smooth muscle contraction. "

To induce asthma, researchers sensitized female mice intraperitoneally—injection into the peritoneal cavity—twice with ovalbumin (OVA) and alum followed by 3 weekly intratracheal challenges with OVA. Allergic airway responses were studied. The now-asthmatic females were treated with ASHMI for 6 weeks, and controls were left untreated. Naïve females constituted an additional control group. The females were then mated with naïve males. Twelve-day-old offspring from each group received 3 consecutive daily intranasal OVA challenges. Two days later, offspring were sacrificed and bronchoalveolar lavage (BAL) *[1] and lung histology were performed. Serum OVA antibodies and cytokine profiles were also assessed. Following the third challenge, total numbers of BAL macrophages, eosinophils, lymphocytes, and neutrophils in the asthmatic but untreated offspring were significantly higher than in BAL of offspring of naïve mothers. The offspring of untreated asthmatic mothers also contained many airway mucus cells. In contrast, the BAL cells from offspring of mothers who had received ASHMI treatment were essentially the same as those of their mothers, no mucus cells were present, and the cytokine profiles were essentially healthy. ASHMI also " significantly suppressed Th2 cytokine

了"对哮喘的主要致病机制(气道高反应性、肺部炎症和气道重塑)以及下调 Th2 反应和直接调节气道平滑肌收缩具有广泛的治疗作用。"

为了诱导哮喘,研究人员通过向雌性小鼠腹腔内注射两次卵白蛋白(OVA)和明矾,然后每周3次气管内注射 OVA 进行致敏。随后,研究气道过敏反应。对现在气喘的雌性小鼠进行6周的 ASHMI 治疗,对照组不作任何处理。未处理雌性小鼠构成另一个对照组。然后,雌性小鼠与未处理雄性小鼠进行交配。从各组中选出12日龄的幼鼠,然后每天接受鼻内 OVA 刺激,连续3天。两天后,幼鼠死去,然后进行支气管肺泡灌洗(BAL)和肺组织学分析。接着,测定血清 OVA 抗体和细胞因子结构。第三次刺激后,未经治疗的哮喘雌性小鼠幼鼠的 BAL 巨噬细胞、嗜酸性粒细胞、淋巴细胞和中性粒细胞的总数明显高于未处理雌性小鼠的幼鼠。未经治疗的哮喘雌性小鼠的幼鼠也含有许多气道黏液细胞。相比而言,经 ASHMI 治疗的雌性小鼠幼鼠的 BAL 细胞与该雌性小鼠的 BAL 细胞基本保持一致,未观察到黏液细胞,并且细胞因子结构也正常。ASHMI 也"显著抑制哮喘患者

---

[1] A bronchoscope is passed into the lungs. Fluid is squirted into the lungs and then collected for study.

支气管窥镜通过肺。液体注射入肺,然后采集液体进行研究。

production by human PBMCs from patients with asthma. "①

A 2011 study② presents explicit suggestion of the epigenetic effects of ASHMI. A group of OVA-allergic-asthmatic female mice were treated with either ASHMI, dexamethasone（a corticosteroid widely used to control asthma）, or water（sham）for 7 weeks. Genomic DNA isolated from lung tissues, collected immediately and 8 weeks post therapy, was bisulfite converted and amplified using polymer-chain-reaction（PCR）technology to study methylation within IFN-γ and IL-4 promoters through pyrosequencing.

Immediately following therapy, methylation at the IFN- promoter was significantly decreased in ASHMI group as compared to sham groups, and to the steroid-group lung tissues, whereas methylation in the IL-4 promoter was significantly increased when compared to the steroid group. The decreases in methylation persisted for at least 8 weeks post therapy. Methylation of CpG at the IL-4 promoter in the lungs of the ASHMI group was significantly higher than in the steroid group. They conclude: " ASHMI resets epigenetic modulation of *IFN*-γ and *IL*-4 expression which is favorable for long-term tolerance induction. "

A subsequent experiment③ examining food allergy instead of allergic asthma used B-FAHF-2 as the

的外周血单核细胞产生 Th2 细胞因子"。

2011 年的一项研究对 ASHMI 的表观遗传效应提出了明确建议。一组 OVA 过敏气喘的雌性小鼠,采用 ASHMI、地塞米松（皮质类固醇,用于控制哮喘）或水（假治疗组）治疗七周,分别于治疗结束后和治疗结束后 8 周收集肺组织的基因组 DNA,采用聚合酶链式反应（PCR）技术进行亚硫酸氢盐转换、扩增,通过焦磷酸测序研究 IFN-γ 和 IL-4 启动子的甲基化。

治疗结束后,立即与假治疗组和类固醇组肺组织相比,ASHMI 组小鼠的 IFN 启动子的甲基化显著降低;然而,与类固醇组相比,在 IL-4 启动子的甲基化显著增加。治疗后甲基化的降低至少持续八周。ASHMI 组小鼠肺组织中的 IL-4 启动子的 CpG 甲基化显著高于类固醇组。他们得出结论:"ASHMI 重置了 IFN-γ 和 IL-4 表达的表观遗传调解,有利于长期的耐受诱导。"

在随后的实验中,采用 B-FAHF-2 作为保护剂,检查食物过敏而不是过敏性哮喘,该保护剂还添加了附加

① Ming-Chun W, et al. Efficacy and tolerability of anti-asthma herbal medicine intervention in adult patients with moderate-severe allergic asthma[J]. Journal of Allergy and Clinical Immunology, 2005, 116(3): 517−524.

② Li X, Srivastava K, Chen J. ASHMI, but not corticosteroid treatment restores maternal allergen long-term tolerance and prevents offspring asthma risk via epigenetic modulation[J]. Journal of Allergy and Clinical Immunology, 2012, 129(2): AB365.

③ Olga, Ying S, Kamal S, et al. The potential of maternal dietary modification for prevention of food allergy[J]. Journal of Allergy & Therapy, 2013(S3): 5.

protective agent with the additional element of determining whether there might also be some benefit with egg allergy, as 70% of peanut-sensitive infants are also sensitive to egg. As before, female mice were sensitized with peanut, then treated with B-FAHF-2 or sham and mated with naïve males. At 5 weeks, offspring were sensitized with egg white and cholera toxin epicutaneously (injections into the skin) 3 times, a week apart. Offspring of mothers that received sham treatment before conception showed significantly higher egg-specific IgE levels than those of naïve mothers. The offspring of B-FAHF-2-treated mothers showed significant suppression of egg-specific IgE compared to the offspring of sham-treated mothers and were essentially the same as naïve offspring.

These results suggest that in addition to its potential as a therapeutic botanical drug, B-FAHF-2 may also have potential for treating food-allergic women prior to conception.

Unfortunately, further investigations of this kind are limited by bias against novelty both for funding and publication. Funding for basic research is generally directed at cures, not prevention. Journals prefer to publish research conducted in discrete steps rather than big leaps, even when those leaps can be convincingly engineered into the scope of an experiment.

Predicting Transmission of Food Allergies

Although maternal allergies are considered a risk factor for food allergies in the next generation, the mechanism is unknown; however, new mouse research

成分可用于测定是否对鸡蛋过敏也有疗效,因为70%的花生过敏婴幼儿也对鸡蛋过敏。同之前一样,雌性小鼠进行花生致敏,经 B-FAHF-2 或假治疗,然后与未处理雄性小鼠交配。第五周时对小鼠生产的幼鼠进行致敏处理,即进行皮下注射注入皮下组织鸡蛋清和霍乱毒素3次,每次间隔一周。在怀孕前接受假治疗的雌性小鼠的幼鼠,其鸡蛋特异性 IgE 水平显著高于未治疗雌性小鼠的幼鼠。接受 B-FAHF-2 治疗的雌性小鼠的幼鼠,与接受假治疗的雌性小鼠的幼鼠相比,其对鸡蛋特异性 IgE 有显著抑制作用,与未处理小鼠的幼鼠相当。

结果表明,B-FAHF-2 除了可以作为治疗性植物药物,也有可能在女性怀孕之前治愈她们的食物过敏症。

不幸的是,由于对新奇研究的偏见,在这方面的进一步研究还受到资金和论文发表的限制。用于基础研究的资金一般是直接用于治疗,而不是预防。而学术期刊更愿意发表以不连续步骤而不是以几次较大的跳跃方式进行的研究,即使这几次较大跳跃能够令人信服地设计在实验范围之内。

预测食物过敏的遗传

尽管母性遗传过敏被视为后代食物过敏的危险因素,但是其机制尚不清楚;然而,宋颖等人进行的新小

by Ying Song et al,[1] points to the chance that heritability of food allergies can be predicted. Five-week-old offspring of peanut-allergic mothers were sensitized with peanut and cholera toxin for 4 weeks, then challenged with peanut. Sensitized offspring of naïve mothers served as a control. They were assessed for anaphylactic reactions, peanut-specific IgE in their blood, and splenocyte and mesenteric MLN cell production of IFN-γ, IL-4, IL-5, IL-10, and IL-17. In addition, the extent of gene expression—CpG methylation—of the IL-4 promoter gene in the offspring's MLN cells was measured. Methylation is a mechanism to regulate how specific genes in the DNA helix do different things at different times (gene expression), as mentioned in the first chapter.

Offspring of the peanut-allergic mothers exhibited significantly higher IgE levels at week 4, as well as more symptoms and lower core body temperature post challenge compared to offspring of normal mothers. Their lymph cells produced significantly more Th2 cytokines and fewer Th1 cytokines than cells from offspring of normal mothers. Reduced methylation at IL-4 promoter was also found. Dr. Song told me that high methylization at a couple of specific sites on the IL-4 gene has now been linked with 90% certainty of allergenicity in offspring. If there were a safe way to treat these mothers who are likely to transmit food allergy epigenetics to their children, it might be possible to reverse the transmission of allergies.

鼠研究指出一种可能性,即预测食物过敏的遗传可能性。花生过敏雌性小鼠生产的 5 周龄幼鼠经花生和霍乱毒素致敏 4 周,之后用花生进行刺激。未处理雌性小鼠生产的过敏幼鼠作为对照。然后,评估它们的过敏反应,它们血液中的花生特异性 IgE,以及脾细胞和肠系膜的 MLN 细胞中 IFN-γ、IL-4、IL-5、IL-10 和 IL-17 的产生水平。此外,测定鼠生产的幼鼠 MLN 细胞中的 IL-4 启动子基因表达程度——CpG 甲基化。甲基化是一种可以调节 DNA 螺旋状物中的特异性基因在不同时间进行不同的基因表达的机制,如第一篇所述。

到第 4 周,与正常雌性小鼠生产的幼鼠相比,花生过敏雌性小鼠生产的幼鼠体内的 IgE 水平显著提高,并且刺激之后它们表现出更多的症状,而它们的核心体温也更低。它们的淋巴细胞产生的 Th2 细胞因子显著高于正常雌性小鼠生产的幼鼠,而其 Th1 细胞因子显著低于正常雌性小鼠生产的幼鼠。同时发现 IL-4 启动子甲基化也减弱了。宋博士告诉我,现在已经确定 IL-4 启动子的数个特定部位的高甲基化与小鼠幼鼠中 90% 的致敏性有关。如果有一种安全的治疗方式可以治愈可能将食物过敏通过表观遗传传递给后代的母亲,就有可能完全逆转过敏症的遗传。

---

[1] Ying S, Ching-feng H, Changda L, et al. Maternal transmission of peanut allergy susceptibility is associated with IL-4 promoter demethylation in offspring[J]. Journal of Allergy and Clinical Immunology, 2013, 131(2): AB218.

Replicating in women the process of low-dosing mice with adjuvant cholera toxin is fraught with ethical and practical obstacles, to say the least, but what if a derivative of cholera toxin could be employed that retained the binding abilities of the full toxin without the toxic effects?

As it happens, there is such a thing. A subunit of cholera toxin called cholera toxin-B (CTB) is the component that first binds to the mucosa. It is considered "an efficient mucosal carrier molecule for the generation of immune responses to linked antigens," with the added benefit that it possesses immunosuppressing qualities of its own.[1] Other researchers learned this the hard way when they tried to induce peanut allergies in mice using CTB instead of cholera toxin and it didn't work. Dr. Li says, "This gave us a clue that CTB might induce tolerance."

One of the studies was "Peanut Tolerance in Offspring of Female Mice Fed Peanut and Cholera Toxin B Subunit Is Associated with Epigenetic Regulation of Foxp3 Promoter and Induction of Mucosal Foxp3 and IL-10 Gene Expression" by Yiqun Hui, Ying Song, and others from Mount Sinai, which was presented at the AAAAI meetings in February of 2013. Dr. Kari Nadeau of Stanford calls Foxp3 genes "peacekeeping" cells and says that children lacking them have more severe allergies, asthma, gastrointestinal diseases, and type-1 diabetes than children with lower levels.[2] IL-10 is an important

退一步说，最起码，在女性身上复制给小鼠服用低剂量佐剂霍乱的过程就充满了伦理和实践障碍。但如果可以使用霍乱毒素的衍生物来保留完整毒素的结合能力，而不产生毒性影响呢？

当它发生时，就会出现这样的事情。称为 CTB 的霍乱毒素亚基可以与黏膜结合。它被视为"一种有效的黏膜载体分子，有助于相关抗原产生免疫反应"，并且它本身具有抑制免疫反应的特点。其他研究人员都知道，当他们试图采用 CTB 代替霍乱毒素诱导小鼠花生过敏时，根本不起作用。李秀敏博士说："这给我们提供了一条线索，即，CTB 可能诱导耐受性。"

其中一项研究是"喂食花生和霍乱毒素亚基的雌性小鼠生产的幼鼠的花生耐受性与 Foxp3 启动子的表观遗传调整以及黏膜 Foxp3 和 IL-10 基因表达的诱导"，作者是西奈山医院的惠益群、宋颖等人，这项研究是 2013 年 2 月在美国过敏、哮喘和免疫学会会议上提交的。斯坦福大学的卡利·纳多博士将 Foxp3 基因称为"维和"细胞，他说，与低水平 Foxp3 基因的儿童相比，缺乏 Foxp3 基因的儿童会患有更严重的过敏、哮喘、胃肠

---

① Antonella D'A, et al. Cholera toxin B subunit promotes the induction of regulatory T cells by preventing human dendritic cell maturation[J]. Journal of Leukocyte Biology, 2008, 84(3): 661－668.

② http://www.asthmaallergies-children.com/2012/09/2 1/turning-the-tables-on-an-%E2%80%9C evolutionary-mistake % E2 % 80% 9D- % E2 % 80 %93-stanford- researchers-go-for-the-cure/.

immunoregulator in the digestive tract and inhibits synthesis of certain inflammatory cytokines. [1]

Having previously reported that maternal consumption of peanut plus nontoxic CTB during pregnancy and subsequent lactation induced tolerance to peanut in mouse offspring, they investigated the potential association of epigenetic changes for inducing tolerance.

Peanut-allergic female mice were either fed low doses of peanut plus CTB or sham-treated during pregnancy and lactation. Intestines were collected from these and naïve offspring. Through a process called quantitative PCR, Foxp3 and IL-10 gene expression were analyzed. DNA methylation of the Foxp3 promoter region was analyzed by bisulfite sequencing PCR. Data were analyzed using one-way ANOVA followed by Bonferroni's tests (statistical methods for excluding random results).

Levels of intestinal IL-10 gene expression were significantly higher in peanut-tolerant offspring than in the allergic and naïve offspring. Intestinal Foxp3 expression in the peanut-tolerant offspring also rose compared to naïve and peanut-allergic ones, respectively. Analysis of DNA methylation revealed decreased methylation levels at the CpG250 Foxp3 promoter site in intestines from the tolerant offspring compared to allergic and naïve offspring. No differences were detected at the other 4 CpG sites.

道疾病以及 I 型糖尿病。IL-10 是消化道中的重要免疫调节剂，它能抑制某些炎性细胞因子的合成。

之前已报道了雌性小鼠在妊娠期和随后的哺乳期摄入花生与无毒霍乱毒素亚基诱导了小鼠后代对花生的耐受性，他们研究了表观遗传变化与诱导耐受性之间的潜在联系。

在花生过敏雌性小鼠的怀孕和哺乳期间，喂食低剂量的花生和无毒霍乱毒素亚基或进行假治疗。收集这些小鼠和未处理小鼠生产的幼鼠的肠道。通过定量聚合酶链式反应分析 Foxp3 和 IL-10 基因表达。通过亚硫酸盐测序聚合酶链式反应分析 Foxp3 启动子区域的 DNA 甲基化。使用单因素方差分析以及邦费罗尼校正（排除随机结果的统计学方法）分析数据。

花生耐受幼鼠中的肠 IL-10 基因表达水平明显高于过敏小鼠和未处理小鼠生产的幼鼠。分别与未处理小鼠和花生过敏小鼠生产幼鼠相比，花生耐受小鼠生产幼鼠中的肠 Foxp3 表达水平也提高了。DNA 甲基化分析显示，在花生耐受小鼠生产的幼鼠的小肠中，CpG250 Foxp3 启动子位点的甲基化水平低于过敏和未处理小鼠生产的幼鼠的甲基化水平。在其他 4 个 CpG 位点，未检测到不同。

[1] http://en. wikipedia. org/wiki/Interleukin_10.

The team concluded that CTB as an adjuvant for peanut immunotherapy appears to be effective and safe in generating oral tolerance in the offspring of sensitized mice.

Given the safety of CTB and the success of inducing tolerance in new generations of mice, this approach holds the prospect of a sea change in the allergy epidemic. Dr. Li says, "Ying's data support our hypothesis. If we can desensitize the allergic mother safely, we may be able to provide trans-generational benefits. We believe this is important because it may be able to reverse the peanut-allergy epidemic."

If this research pans out, fewer mothers will ask the question, "What did I do wrong?"

⑭ Beyond Food Allergies

One of the more tantalizing aspects of Dr. Li's work is its potential for treating conditions beyond allergies. Though allergies have proliferated in populations around the world, for people who don't have them or whose allergies can be minimized with relatively inexpensive measures, allergies don't sound like public enemy number one. Disordered immunity has now been linked to a much wider set of noncommunicable diseases (NCDs) that raise more eyebrows, and indeed more money, than allergies, however. Allergies may function as a kind of early warning system for NCDs, like a canary in a coal mine. Dr. Susan Prescott says, "(A)s the most common and earliest-onset NCD, the epidemic of allergic diseases points to specific vulnerability of the developing immune system to modern environmental change. Indeed, many environmental risk factors implicated in the rise of other NCDs have been shown to mediate their effects through

该研究小组得出的结论是,无毒霍乱毒素亚基作为花生免疫疗法的佐剂,在致敏小鼠生产的幼鼠中产生口服耐受似乎是有效安全的。

考虑到无毒霍乱毒素亚基的安全性和在新一代小鼠的诱导耐受的成功,这种方法有望给过敏流行治疗带来巨大的变化。李秀敏博士说:"宋颖的数据支持了我们的假设。如果我们可以安全地使过敏的母亲脱敏,那么我们可能能够提供跨代效益。我们相信这是重要的,它或许能够扭转花生过敏流行病。"

如果本研究取得成功,会有更少的母亲问"我做错了什么?"

⑭ 应用于食物过敏之外的疾病的可能

李秀敏博士的工作更令人兴奋的一个方面是治疗除了过敏以外的其他病症的潜力。尽管过敏在全世界人口中扩散,对于没有过敏或可以通过相对廉价措施减轻过敏的人们而言,过敏听起来不像是头号公敌。目前,紊乱免疫与一系列更广泛的令人吃惊的非传染性疾病(NCDs)有关,这些疾病比过敏更让人费脑筋和费钱。过敏对于非传染性疾病起到一种预警系统的作用,就好像矿井里的金丝雀一样。苏珊·普莱斯考特博士说:"作为最常见和最早发病的非传染性疾病,过敏性疾病的流行表明发展中的免疫系统对现代环境变化的特殊脆弱性。事实上,许多与其

immune pathways." Put another way, if environmental changes are doing this much damage to people who have allergies, isn't it reasonable to suppose that they might be hurting the nonallergic in other ways?

Dr. Prescott writes, "The innate immune system provides a clear example of this convergence, with evidence that physical activity, nutrition, pollutants, and the microbiome all influence systemic inflammation through Toll-like receptor pathways (notably Toll-like receptor 4), with downstream effects on the risk of insulin resistance, obesity, cardiovascular risk, immune diseases, and even mood and behavior."[1]

Dr. Renata Engler is also intrigued by this thesis. She commented in notes to me after reviewing the manuscript of this book:

The growing evidence that chronic inflammation is a key player in the major killer diseases is I believe a major 21st century medicine paradigm shift. The hypothesis that allergic individuals may have an increased risk for cardiovascular disease has yet to be tested but is a strong candidate. Chronic sinusitis and periodontal disease increase risk of cardiovascular disease; there is considerable evidence in the literature for this. Integrative medicine approaches to cardiovascular disease prevention include careful attention to dental health, underlying sources of chronic infection and inflammation. The non-specific

他非传染性疾病上升有关的环境风险因素已被证明可以通过免疫途径介导其影响。"换言之,如果环境改变对患有过敏症的人群伤害较大,是否可以合理推断环境改变以其他方式伤害非过敏人群?

普莱斯考特博士写道:"先天免疫系统为这种趋同提供了明显的例子。证据表明体育活动、营养物、污染物和微生物组均可通过 Toll 样受体途径(尤其是 Toll 样受体 4)影响全身性炎症。对胰岛素抗性、肥胖、心血管风险和免疫疾病,甚至是情绪和行为,都具有负面影响。"

勒娜特·恩格勒博士也对本书很感兴趣。审查完本书的手稿之后,她写下评注:

越来越多的证据表明,慢性炎症是主要致命疾病的关键因素,我相信,这是 21 世纪主要的医学范式转换。过敏人群患心血管疾病的风险增加的假设尚未得到证实,但它是一个重要的潜在因素。慢性鼻窦炎和牙周病会增加患心血管疾病的风险,在医学文献中对此具有相当多的证据。心血管疾病预防的中西医结合方法包括仔细注意保持牙周健康、预防慢性感染和炎症的潜在来源。被

① Susan L P. Early-Life environmental determinants of allergic diseases and the wider pandemic of inflammatory noncommunicable diseases[J]. Journal of Allergy and Clinical Immunology, 2013, 131(1): 23-30.

marker of inflammation known as C-reactive protein (CRP) is a biomarker of cardiovascular inflammation risk with hyperlipidemia. Better drugs are needed to downregulate inflammation without undermining appropriate immune defenses. What if the TCM therapies that have shown such potential in modulating the immune system for treating allergies could also be applied to other conditions?

In a book called *The Genius Within：Discovering the Intelligence of Every Living Thing*, author Frank T. Vertosick Jr. wrote, "The immune system must learn and recall billions, perhaps trillions, of different molecular patterns. Our lives depend on its ability to make instant discriminations between friend and foe, not an easy task." That capability is a wondrous thing, but when it goes wrong, it is also terrifying. The huge cast of T cells, B cells, mast cells, basophils, and the cytokines that regulate their behavior are like a stock company in a series of dramas. In a person with intestinal parasites, IgE wears a white hat and plays the hero. In a food allergy patient, it wears a black hat and plays the villain. We need treatments that can modulate excesses and insufficiencies without creating new problems. To paraphrase Dr. Li, we want to make bad boys into good boys without turning good girls bad.

The growing database of herbs that Dr. Li is compiling at Mount Sinai provides an intriguing foundation for new generations of potential treatments for a broad range of diseases. In making the leap from intestinal parasites to food allergies, Dr. Li found a treatment that seems to work, but in exploring the underlying biochemistry, trying to find out why it

称为炎症的非特异性标记 C 反应蛋白（CRP）是含有高脂血心血管炎症风险的生物标记。在不损害适当的免疫防御情况下，需要使用较好的药物使消炎。在调节免疫系统治疗过敏中表现得很有潜力的中药，如果用于其他病症，会怎样呢？

法兰克·佛杜锡克在《内在的天才：发现万物的智慧》一书中写道："免疫系统必须学习并回忆数十亿或者数万亿不同的分子模型。我们的生命依赖于它能即时鉴定朋友和敌人的能力，而这不是一个简单的任务。"这种能力是一件很奇妙的事情，但是当它出错时，也是非常可怕的。调节自身行为的大量的 T 细胞、B 细胞、肥大细胞、嗜碱性粒细胞和调节它们行为的细胞因子犹如一系列电视剧中的一个股份公司。在有肠道寄生虫的患者身上，IgE 头戴白帽子，扮演英雄。在食物过敏患者身上，它头戴黑帽，扮演坏人。在不引起新问题的情况下，我们需要调节过度和不足的治疗方法。引用李秀敏博士的意思，我们想将坏男孩变成好男孩，而不是将好女孩变成坏女孩。

李秀敏博士在西奈山医院编写的不断增长的草药数据库为新一代的广泛疾病的潜在治疗方法提供了有趣的基础。从肠道寄生虫到食物过敏的飞跃中，李秀敏博士发现了一个似乎有效的治愈方法，但是在探索潜在的生物化学，并试图发现它为什

works, she found clues to possible shortcuts for treatment of diseases that are non-allergic but that also entail malfunctions of the immune system.

Several projects now underway at Sinai demonstrate the possibilities for treating debilitating diseases without the destructive side effects that accompany conventional immune suppression.

I am reporting these experiments not because they represent the prospect of any immediate breakthroughs across a broad spectrum of diseases. Exciting though the experiments are, the odds are against success. My great friend Dr. Mark Cullen of Stanford, who read this manuscript, got hung up on this point:

I am always a little leery of the wistful "look how far this could go" speculation, which has become taboo in scientific writing. Since every single biologic process is tied to a trillion others, speculation about how control of one pathway might positively influence others is tempting, but it almost never pans out when challenged. The sections on Crohn's and cancer are too great a leap—I doubt Dr. Li will make contributions to those fields, sorry, and may tempt readers to draw the wrong conclusions. Asthma looks far more likely to bear fruit, but you'd be amazed how wrong most such speculations have proved to be historically. Ask any friend in pharma R&D!

Thank you, Dr. Cullen. And I wouldn't be amazed.

With Mark's admonition in mind, I'd like to point out that whatever happens may well yield greater

么有效的过程中,她发现了一些线索,可能是治疗非过敏疾病的快捷方式,但是该方法也导致免疫系统功能发生障碍。

西奈山医院正在进行的几个项目证明了在常规免疫抑制不产生破坏性副作用的情况下,治疗衰竭性疾病的可能性。

我报道这些实验并不是因为它们代表了在广泛的疾病领域即将取得突破的前景。尽管这些实验令人兴奋,但成功的概率是不大的。我的好朋友,斯坦福大学的马克·卡伦博士读完本手稿后,就这一点十分担忧:

我总是对渴望"看它能够走多远"的推测有点怀疑,这已成为科学写作中的禁忌。因为每个单一生物过程与一万亿其他生物过程相连,关于控制一个途径如何对其他途径产生积极影响的猜测很有吸引力。但是当挑战时,几乎从来都不成功。有关克罗恩病和癌症的章节(和过敏相比)跳跃太大了——我怀疑李秀敏博士是否能对这些领域作出贡献,抱歉,这可能会诱使读者得出错误的结论。治疗哮喘似乎更有可能取得成果,但你会惊讶地发现,历史上大多数这样的推测已证明是大错特错。问问制药研发领域的朋友!

谢谢你,卡伦博士。我没有感到惊讶。

考虑到马克的告诫,我想指出的是,无论发生什么,都很可能让我们对起作用的生理机制有更深入的了

insight into the physiological mechanisms at work. Dr. Sicherer at Mount Sinai said that Dr. Li's research has already taught us things about the immune system.

The Western pharmacopoeia is full of botanical derivatives that do work, which is one of the reasons that biodiversity is so critical. Who knows what matches remain to be made between in the molecules of herbs and flowers on one continent and the T cells of sick individuals on another? The classical physicians of China did a lot of research and development for us. They showed us that certain botanicals work for certain things. Contemporary scientists can show us how those botanicals work, and by doing so, they give us clues to still other applications.

▌Inflammatory Bowel Disease

Among the doctors who are now collaborating with Dr. Li is David Dunkin, a gastroenterologist at Mount Sinai who spends four days a week doing research and one day mainly treating young patients with Crohn's disease and ulcerative colitis, which fall under the umbrella of inflammatory bowel disease. They have similar symptoms to one another— abdominal pain, rectal bleeding, diarrhea, weight loss, fever, and skin and eye involvement—but they differ in the way they affect different parts of the intestinal tract. [1]

Crohn's has been a focal point of research at Sinai for many decades and is named for gastroenterologist Dr. Burrill Bernard Crohn, who worked there. In 1932, working with two other colleagues, Crohn described a series of patients with inflammation of the

解。西奈山的史可瑞博士说,李秀敏博士的研究已经教会了我们一些有关免疫系统的知识。

西方药典包含了有效的植物制成品,这是生物多样性如此至关重要的原因之一。谁知道在一个大陆的草药和花朵分子与另一个大陆的患病个体的 T 细胞之间存在什么样的配对?传统中医为我们做了大量的研究和开发。他们向我们展示了某些植物性治疗药物对某些疾病起作用。当代科学家可向我们展示那些植物性治疗药物是如何起作用的,通过这样来做,他们还为我们提供了其他应用方面的线索。

▌炎症性肠病

目前与李秀敏博士合作的医生中有一位是来自西奈山医院的胃肠病学家大卫·邓金。他每周花费四天的时间从事研究工作,并花费一天的时间治疗患有克罗恩病和溃疡性结肠炎的年轻患者,这些患者属于炎症性肠炎疾病患者。他们具有类似的症状,例如腹痛、直肠出血、腹泻、体重减轻、发烧以及皮肤和眼部损害,但是其影响肠道不同部位的方式不同。

几十年来,克罗恩病一直是西奈山医院的研究热点之一,并且是以在那工作的胃肠病学家伯里尔·伯纳德·克罗恩博士命名的。1932 年,克罗恩和另外两个同事一起,描述了一系列患有末端回肠炎的患者,末端

---

① http://ibdcrohns.about.com/ cs/ibdfaqs/ a/ibdl 01 . htm.

terminal ileum, the area most commonly affected by the illness. ① Dunkin says that he can diagnose Crohn's children very quickly because they are characteristically very pale, thin, and below average in growth. Failure to thrive is common.

Crohn's is considered an autoimmune disease. The roster of cytokines with which you are now familiar from earlier chapters may be directed at any tissue between the esophagus and the rectum, resulting in chronic destructive inflammation. As with food allergies, there is no cure, although Crohn's and colitis can be held in check by blocking the production of cytokines and suppressing inflammation with steroids. The trouble with these remedies, however, is that, as is the case with allergies, they are very blunt instruments. Systemic steroids block good cytokines along with bad and can have a debilitating effect on defenses against infections.

For children with active disease, life isn't much fun. "They have to stay home or in the hospital and typically take these strong medicines three times a day," says Dunkin. "And with chronic symptoms like diarrhea, they don't much feel like being around other kids."

Dunkin's research took a new direction when Dr. Li called him and pointed out that her research showed that FAHF-2 inhibited production of TNF-α, which was discussed in chapters 6 and 11. Dr. Li knew that high levels of TNF-α were also associated with Crohn's. According to Bellantd et al, TNF-α increases

回肠是最常患病的区域。邓金说他可以很快地诊断出克罗恩病患儿,因为他们的特征是苍白、瘦弱,生长发育低于平均水平,而且通常无法茁壮成长。

克罗恩病被视为一种自体免疫性疾病。从前面的章节中我们已经熟悉的细胞因子可指向食道和直肠之间的任何组织,从而导致慢性破坏性炎症。尽管克罗恩病和结肠炎可以通过阻止细胞因子生产并用类固醇抑制炎症,但正如食物过敏一样,是没有治愈方法的。然而,就像过敏一样,这些疗法的问题是它们是非常生硬的手段。全身性类固醇会阻断好的以及坏的细胞因子,并极大地削弱防御感染能力。

对于过敏活跃期患儿而言,生活没有太多的乐趣。邓金博士说:"他们不得不待在家里或医院,并且要服用这些强效药,一天三次。对于患有慢性症状如腹泻的患儿而言,他们不喜欢和其他孩子一起玩耍。"

当李秀敏博士打电话给邓金并指出她的研究表明 FAHF-2 抑制了 TNF-α 的产生时,邓金的研究换了一个新的研究方向,这在第 6 篇和第 11 篇中有所讨论。李秀敏博士知道,高水平的 TNF-α 与克罗恩病有

---

① http://en.wikipedia.org/wiki/Crohn%27s_disease.

the transport of white blood cells to inflamed sites and activates neutrophils and eosinophils. [1] This induces tissue-degrading enzymes, the results of which are visible to anyone who sees endoscopic photographs of ulcers of the affected tissue. They look to me like what would happen to your skin if you rubbed it with sandpaper.

Dr. Li and Dr. Dunkin discussed whether it was possible to modulate the immune system for Crohn's as had been case with food allergies. He took blood and gut tissue samples from new patients who had been diagnosed but not yet treated, and he examined the samples for the cytokines they produced. When FAHF-2 was added to these tissues, the inflammatory cytokines were reduced.

In vitro research has since confirmed the modulating effects of FAHF-2 for Crohn's patients as well as allergic ones, and a mouse study has also had encouraging results. Dunkin says that his research has excited patients. "They ask how the Chinese study is going, but I have to caution them it will be years before there's any realistic prospect of treatment."

Note: A clinical study described as follows, is now underway at Mount Sinai:

The purpose of this study is to see if inflammatory cytokines (markers or chemicals in the blood/tissue that are associated with active inflammatory bowel disease) will be affected by the addition of Chinese herbal medicines that are added to cultures of blood cells or tissue specimens from the colon. A blood sample will

关。根据 Bellantd 等人的研究，TNF-α 加速了白细胞向发炎部位的运输，并激活了中性粒细胞和嗜酸性粒细胞。这诱导了组织降解酶，其结果对于任何看到患病组织的溃疡的内镜照片的人都是可见的。在我看来，这就像你用砂纸摩擦你的皮肤会发生的状况。

李秀敏博士和邓金博士讨论了是否有可能像治疗食物过敏那样调节克罗恩病的免疫系统。他采集血样、收集已确诊但未治疗的新患者的肠道组织样本，并检查了它们产生的细胞因子样本。当 FAHF-2 添加到这些组织中时，炎性细胞因子减少。

体外研究已证实了 FAHF-2 对克罗恩病患者以及过敏患者的调节作用，一项小鼠研究也取得了令人鼓舞的结果。邓金说他的研究让病人很兴奋。"他们询问中国的研究进展如何，但是我必须提醒要实现任何的治疗前景，需要花费许多年的时间。"

注：以下描述的临床研究正在西奈山医院进行：

本研究的目的是探索炎性细胞因子(血液/组织中的与活动期炎症性肠病相关的标记物或化学物)是否将受到添加到血细胞培养皿或结肠的组织样本培养皿的中草药的添

---

[1] Bellanti J A, et al., op cit.

be drawn at the time of endoscopy. The blood sample will be used to obtain serum and white blood cells. The colonic (taken from the large intestine/colon) sample will be used to obtain tissue cells. [1]

Organ Rejection

One immune disorder that has spawned research under Dr. Li's auspices is very different from any other. Unlike allergies, in which the immune system turns against otherwise innocuous proteins in the environment and diet, or autoimmune diseases, in which the body attacks itself, in this case, the antigen is deliberately introduced for the purposes of saving lives. This represents the supreme contest between modern technical medical capabilities and the best the immune system has to offer—organ transplantation. Without concerted efforts to suppress its action, the immune system regards the new tissue as a massive virus, microbe, or allergen, and sets out to destroy it.

Surgeons have dreamed of transplanting organs and limbs for centuries, but except for corneas, the first successful organ transplant was only done in 1954, a kidney from one identical twin to the other. Because the twins' genes were the same, organ rejection was not an issue.

Transplantation between non-twins would have to wait for the development of immune suppressants that were safe and effective enough to be used daily for a lifetime. Cortisone has too many side effects. It was not until 1970, when cyclosporine was discovered in the fungus *Tolypodadium inflatum*, that surgeons

加物的影响。血样将在内窥镜检查的时候取出。并且,血样将用于获得血清和白细胞。结肠样本(取自大肠/结肠)将用于获得组织细胞。

器官排异

在李秀敏博士主持的一项基于免疫缺陷的研究和其他同类研究差异极大。不同于过敏反应,免疫系统转而抵抗环境和饮食中的其他无害蛋白,自体攻击的免疫性疾病,这种情况是为了挽救生命而故意引入抗原。这代表了现代医疗技术能力和免疫系统发挥最大效用之间的最强的竞争——器官移植。(器官移植是)未经两者共同作用下的行为,免疫系统会将新的组织视为大规模的病毒、细菌或过敏原,并开始摧毁它。

几个世纪以来,外科医生一直梦想着移植器官和四肢。但除了角膜之外,第一次成功的器官移植于1954年完成,是一对同卵双胞胎间的肾脏移植。因为双胞胎的基因是相同的,所以器官排异不是问题。

非双胞胎之间的移植只能等待免疫抑制剂的开发,这些抑制剂要足够安全有效且可以一生中每天使用。可的松具有太多的副作用。直到1970年,当环孢霉素在真菌Tolypodadium inflatum中被发现时,

---

[1] http://icahn. mssm. edu/research/programs/jaffe-food-allergy-insti- tute/clinical-trials.

acquired a medication suitable to make transplantation the relatively commonplace procedure it has become. Another drug, sirolimus/rapamycin was first found in the bacterium *Streptomyces hygroscopicus* on Easter Island. ①

Although better post-transplantation clinical care and a larger repertoire of immunosuppression approaches have reduced short-term illness and lowered rates of acute organ rejection, these remain a persistent threat. Moreover, immunosuppressant drugs can cause a range of toxic side effects. ②

Adapting an ancient herbal preparation to procedures that have been tenable for only 40 years may seem unlikely, but Dr. Jessica Reid-Adam has been exploring this possibility for several years in collaboration with Dr. Peter Heeger, her mentor at Mount Sinai and a transplant immunologist, and Dr. Li.

Dr. Reid-Adam is a pediatric nephrologist. That is, she specializes in kidney disease in children and spends much of her time treating end-stage renal failure. Her typical patient, or patient's parents, face just three choices—dying, dialysis, or transplant. Of these, transplantation is the best, in her estimation. "Dialysis means spending hours being hooked up to a machine at a dialysis center three times a week. There is home dialysis, but it requires a certain amount of room and a good deal of discipline."

外科医生才获得一种适合于使移植成为相对常见的手术的药物。另一种药物,西罗莫司/雷帕霉素在复活节岛的吸水链霉菌中首次被发现。

尽管更好的移植术后临床护理和更多的免疫抑制方法减少了短期疾病发生并降低了急性器官排异的发生率,但是,这些仍然是持续存在的威胁。此外,免疫抑制药物可引起一系列毒副作用。

让一种古老的草药制剂适用于仅有40年历史的手术似乎不太可能,但是在过去的几年中,杰西卡·里德·亚当博士与她在西奈山医院的导师彼得·黑格博士,一位移植免疫学家,还有李秀敏博士的合作已探索了这种可能性。

里德·亚当博士是儿童肾病学家。换言之,她专研儿童肾脏疾病并花费大量时间治疗终末期肾功能衰竭。她的典型的患者或其患者的父母只面临三个选择——死亡、透析或移植。在这三个选择中,她估计移植是最好的方法。"透析意味着花费几个小时连接至透析中心的机器,一周三次。也有在家里进行透析的,但是需要一定的空间,并遵循操作规程。"

---

① http://en.wikipedia.org/wiki/ Organ_transplantation.
② Reid-Adam J, Yang N, Song Y, et al. Immunosuppressive effects of the traditional Chinese herb Qu Mai on human alloreactive T cells[J]. American Journal of Transplantation, 2013, 13(5): 1159 –1167.

When Jessica began her nephrology fellowship after completing training in pediatrics, she didn't have a research agenda. Her ambition was to work with patients, but research was a necessary part of her training. Her fellowship director, Dr. Jeff Saland, had heard Xiu-Min Li give a talk and suggested that Jessica get in touch with Dr. Li to see if there was something in TCM that might be applied in organ transplantation.

"Xiu-Min said she had a database of herbs and that I should see which ones sounded like they might apply to the kidneys," says Reid-Adam.

Transplantation presents a number of terrible challenges, apart from acquiring compatible organs. "Some of our patients are transplanted under the age of two. "

Patients must be closely monitored for any signs of rejection and must take large amounts of immune-suppressing drugs. Moreover, the life expectancy of an individual organ is limited—typically to 5—10 years, although one patient known to Dr. Reid-Adam still has a kidney with no signs of failure after 18 years. "Most of them get an adult organ," she says. "This is not a problem surgically—all the veins and arteries connect. The real difficulty is the immune suppression. An allergy is a reaction to proteins that can be measured in micrograms. A kidney is usually 125 grams or more— 5 ounces of foreign tissue in a child weighing 20 pounds. "

The drugs present an additional problem: " The immune systems of small children are immature. At least an adult has some degree of protection against infection even after their immunity is suppressed.

当杰西卡完成儿科培训后,回到她的肾脏科研究员职位时,她并没有研究计划。她的志向是与患者一起工作,但研究是培训的必要组成部分。她的研究员主任杰夫·萨兰德博士听过李秀敏博士的演讲后,就建议杰西卡与李秀敏博士联系,以观察中药是否可用于器官移植手术中。

里德·亚当说:"秀敏说她有一个草药数据库,并且我应看看哪些听起来像是可能用于肾脏。"

除了获得匹配的器官外,移植还面临着一些可怕的挑战。"我们的一些患者是在两岁以内进行移植的。"

需对患者的任何排异迹象密切监测,并且患者应服用大量免疫抑制药物。此外,单个器官的预期寿命是有限的——通常为 5 ~ 10 年,尽管里德·亚当博士认识的一名患者移植的肾脏在 18 年后仍然没有衰竭迹象。她说:"他们中的大部分获得的是成年人的器官。这不是外科手术问题,手术只需连接所有的静脉和动脉。真正的困难是免疫抑制。过敏是对可以用微克来测量的蛋白质的反应。对于一个体重 20 磅的孩子来说,肾脏通常是 125 克或更多 5 盎司的异物组织。"

该药物呈现出另外的问题:"儿童的免疫系统是不成熟的。即使成年人的免疫被抑制之后,至少还具有某种程度的抗感染保护。儿童没有

Children don't have time to develop this capacity, which makes them even more vulnerable to incidental infection and certain types of cancer."

Also, current immunosuppressants have little or no effect on memory T cells formed to react to the donated tissue, which is problematic because the transplanted organ is always there. The immune response will never go away. As Dr. Reid-Adam and her coauthors say in their first major publication, "Taken together, these observations support the need to identify additional immunosuppressants for use in transplantation, specifically compounds that are simultaneously Treg-protective and capable of blocking memory T cells."[1]

With guidance from Dr. Heeger, Dr. Reid-Adam and her coresearchers screened extracts from 53 traditional Chinese herbs for their ability to suppress human alloreactive T cells (T cells mobilized by the presence of transplanted tissue). The team reasoned that herbs would ideally inhibit production of the proinflammatory cytokine IFN-γ and simultaneously augment production of the immunoregulatory cytokine IL-10. Says Reid-Adam, "An increase in IFN-γ is good for allergies but bad for organ rejection. However, IL-10, which sometimes indicates greater Th2 activity but not really Th1, can be a beneficial indicator for allergies and also good for transplantation."

Employing an *in vitro* version of transplantation—culturing cells from one individual and then exposing those to cells from another—they analyzed the cytokines in the presence of each herb, using the

时间发育这种能力,这使得他们更容易受到感染并患上某种类型的癌症。"

而且,目前的免疫抑制剂对能向移植入组织作出反应的记忆 T 细胞影响很小或没有影响,这是有问题的,因为移植器官会一直存在。免疫反应永远不会消失。正如里德·亚当博士和她的合作者在他们的第一篇主要论文中所述:"总的来说,这些观察结果支持鉴定用于移植的其他免疫抑制剂的需要,尤其是同时保护 Treg 和能够抑制记忆 T 细胞的化合物。"

在黑格博士的指导下,里德·亚当博士和她的共同研究者筛选了能够抑制人类同种异体反应性 T 细胞的 53 种中草药的提取物(T 细胞因移植组织的出现而激活)。该研究小组推断草药将理想地抑制促炎细胞因子 IFN-γ 的产生,并同时增加免疫调节细胞因子 IL-10 的产生。里德·亚当说:"IFN-γ 的增加对过敏是好的,但是对于器官排异是有害的。然而,IL-10 有时表明 Th2 而非 Th1 的活性较高,它可以作为过敏的有益指标,也有利于移植。"

他们采用体外移植的方法——培养一个个体的细胞,然后将这些细胞暴露给另一个个体的细胞——用标准的低剂量—高剂量方案分析每

---

① Ibid p. 1159.

standard low-dose-high-dose protocol.

They identified *Qu Mai* (QM, *Dianthus Superbus*), a member of the carnation family, as a candidate. Dr. Reid-Adam says, "There isn't much written about it in Western literature, but TCM practitioners use it to treat blood in urine and urinary infection, indicating a connection to the kidney, and for skin inflammation. It achieves the decrease in an important proinflammatory cytokine without killing immune cells." Testing in paired doses they found that the higher the dose, the greater improvement in the ratio of IL-10 to IFN-γ.

Further research based on polarity isolated three fractions of active compounds from the QM herbal preparation. These were dichloromethane-soluble QMAD (mainly contains nonpolar compounds), ethyl acetate-soluble QMAE (mainly contains less polar compounds), and butanol-soluble QMAB (mainly contains moderate polar compounds). Testing each fraction for its effects on cytokine production showed that the QMAD fraction induced the most favorable effects, yielding a ninefold increase in IL-10 : IFN-γ ratios.

The QMAD data show an additional benefit over conventional immunosuppressants, which show limited ability to modulate the memory T cells. This in effect keeps the immune system in a state of continuous emergency as long as the foreign tissue remains in the body. The "data show unequivocal effects of QMAD on inhibiting proliferation and IFN-γ production by naïve and memory T cells while simultaneously facilitating Treg induction. The observed ability of QMAD to block proliferation and cytokine secretion by memory T cells is of particular interest, as memory T

种草药中存在的细胞因子。

他们将瞿麦(QM,瞿麦),康乃馨家族的一员,作为候选者。里德·亚当博士说:"西方文献中没有太多有关它的书面描述,但是中医师用它来治疗尿血和尿道感染,表明它与肾脏和皮肤炎症的联系。瞿麦能在不杀死免疫细胞的情况下减少一种重要的促炎细胞因子。"在配对剂量测试中,他们发现剂量越高,IL-10 与 IFN-γ 的比值提高越大。

基于极性的进一步研究,她们从瞿麦草药制剂中分离出三种活性成分。这些混合物为可溶二氯甲烷 QMAD(主要包括非极性化合物)、可溶乙酸乙酯 QMAE(主要包括低极性化合物)以及可溶丁醇 QMAB(主要包括中等极性化合物)。经测试每种活性成分对细胞因子产生的影响表明,QMAD 部分诱导最有利的影响,在 IL-10 与 IFN-γ 比值中产生九倍的增长量。

QMAD 数据表明优于传统免疫抑制剂的额外好处,这显示调节记忆 T 细胞的有限的能力。实际上,只要外来组织仍存在于体内,免疫系统就会保持连续紧急的状态。"有数据表明 QMAD 通过初始和记忆 T 细胞抑制增殖和 IFN-γ 产生的明确效果,并同时促进 Treg 诱导。观察到的QMAD 抑制记忆 T 细胞增殖和细胞因子分泌的能力特别令人感兴趣,因

cells are generally resistant to immunosuppression and have been implicated as key mediators of allograft * [①] injury." If this pans out in subsequent research, it will ease some of the perpetual struggle between the patient's own immune system and the new organ, possibly prolonging the life of each transplanted kidney and improving the patient's quality of life.

Two cautionary notes: As Dr. Cullen points out, favorable test-tube results do not guarantee clinical efficacy, and unlike FAHF-2, Dr. Reid-Adam's work is not likely to lead to a "cure." Assuming QM proves itself in animal models, the population of human subjects whose kidneys are failing can't submit to placebo-controlled trials or be left untreated to test lasting efficacy.

"I see it as adjunctive," Dr. Reid-Adam says. "Anything that can provide relief and mitigate damage from general immune suppression will be a great step forward."

Asthma

Dollar for dollar, and life for life, asthma poses the largest challenge to American public health, and indeed around the world, of any allergic disease. As discussed in chapter 1, asthma takes more than 3,000 lives every year, including almost 200 children under

为记忆 T 细胞通常是抵抗免疫抑制的,并被视为同种异体移植损伤的关键介质。"如果在后续的研究中取得成功,它将缓和患者自身免疫系统和新的器官之间的永久的斗争,可能延长每个移植肾脏的寿命并提高患者的生活质量。

两个警示:正如卡伦博士所指出的,有利的试管结果并不能保证临床疗效,与 FAHF-2 不同,里德·亚当博士的工作不太可能产生"治愈方法"。假设瞿麦在动物模型中证明了自己,但肾脏衰竭的人群无法接受安慰剂对照试验,也无法接受长期疗效测试。

里德·亚当说:"我将其视为辅助疗法,从一般免疫抑制中,任何可以提供缓解并减轻伤害的发现都将是向前迈进的一大步。"

哮喘

考虑到花费的金钱和逝去的生命,哮喘对美国的公共卫生构成了最大的挑战,实际上在世界范围内,任何过敏性疾病都是如此。正如第一篇中所讨论的,哮喘每年夺走 3 000 多人的生命,包括将近 200 名 15 岁

[①] * "Allograft: The transplant of an organ or tissue from one individual to another of the same species with a different genotype. For example, a transplant from one person to another, but not an identical twin, is an allograft. Allografts account for many human transplants, including those from cadaveric, living related, and living unrelated donors." (MedicineNet. com)

"同种异体移植:将一个器官或组织从一个个体移植到另一个具有不同基因型的同种动物身上。例如,从一个人移植到另一个人,但不是同卵双胞胎,是同种异体移植。人体移植大多数是同种异体移植,包括来自尸体、活体亲属和活体非亲属捐赠者的移植。"(MedicineNet. com)

the age of 15. [1] The medical costs and indirect costs such as lost productivity at work and at school come to $ 56 billion annually. Per capita, the burden is even worse in many other countries, including, notably, New Zealand, Australia, and the United Kingdom.

In all these countries, however, mortality rates have fallen considerably with the use of inhaled corticosteroids (ICS) the biggest factor in improvement. Still, many of the continuing deaths are considered preventable, if only more patients were compliant with their medication regimes. Apart from the cost of medication and the day-to-day aggravation of taking medicine, the negative associations with the word " steroids " in the name is a major barrier, although corticosteroids have no connection to the testosterone-based steroids that athletes use.

ASHMI, described in the previous chapter, may present an effective alternative to ICS. In an early double-blind, randomized, placebo-controlled trial investigating the efficacy and tolerability of ASHMI compared with oral prednisone therapy in 91 patients with moderate-to-severe asthma, treatment was administered daily over 4 weeks. [2] After treatment, lung function was significantly improved in both groups, and clinical symptom scores, use of bronchodilators, and serum IgE levels and Th2 cytokine levels were reduced. Unlike prednisone, ASHMI significantly increased serum IFN-γ and cortisol levels while no significant side effects were observed. (Cordsol is the body's own cortisone,

以下的儿童（指在美国，译者注）。医疗费用和间接成本，比如工作和学校的生产力损失，每年总计 560 亿美元。在许多其他国家，尤其是新西兰、澳大利亚和英国，人均负担更重。

然而，在所有这些国家中，死亡率大幅下降，吸入性皮质类固醇（ICS）的使用是改善的最大因素。尽管如此，许多持续的死亡被认为是可以预防的，只要更多的患者按时按量服药。除了药物的成本和每天服用药量的加重，名称中与"类固醇"一词的负面关联是一个主要障碍，尽管皮质类固醇与运动员使用的基于睾酮的类固醇没有联系。

前面章节中所述的 ASHMI 可能是 ICS 的有效替代品。一项早期的双盲、随机安慰剂对照试验，在 4 周内每天进行治疗，研究了 ASHMI 与口服泼尼松治疗的 91 名患有中度至重度哮喘的患者相比的疗效和耐受性。治疗后，两组肺功能明显改善，临床症状评分、支气管扩张药的使用、血清 IgE 水平和 Th2 细胞因子水平均下降。与泼尼松不同，ASHMI 明显提高了血清 IFN-γ 和皮质醇水平，而没有观察到明显的副作用。（皮质醇是身体自身的可的松，

---

[1] "Trends in Asthma Morbidity and Mortality" from American Lung Association, Epidemiology and Statistics Unit, Research and Health Education Division, September 2012.

[2] Wen et al., op cit.

which helps mitigate allergic activity.) Subsequent experiments affirmed safety and tolerance, as well as favorable intermodulatory effects on cytokines, IgE levels, and bronchoconstriction. [1]

Taken together these studies showed that ASHMI was safe and well tolerated in clinical study. ASHMI also showed multiple beneficial effects in allergic asthma. Because ASHMI enhanced IFN-γ, and normalized cortisol levels in a clinical study, future clinical investigations should determine if ASHMI can restore/normal IFN-γ and cortisol levels when used in combination with corticosteroids. Identification of active compounds in ASHMI will enhance our understanding of the pharmacological mechanisms of ASHMI and may lead to novel drugs for asthma therapy. [2]

(ASHMI is not the only TCM-derived asthma treatment under study. A more complete discussion is available in the review article cited above.)

Dr. Li already uses ASHMI in her clinic, where it is used as a supplement rather than a drug. "We have to be careful," she says. "Our eczema treatment can start on day one. With steroids, you can't just suddenly stop and switch to something new because inflammation may return while the new treatment takes hold. We introduce the new treatment and taper off the steroids. The whole time, we keep records on IgE levels and lung function, which confirm what we are

有助于缓解过敏活动。)后续试验确认了安全性和耐受性以及对细胞因子、IgE 水平和支气管收缩的良好的相互调节作用。

综合这些研究表明 ASHMI 在临床研究中是安全的且耐受良好的。在过敏性哮喘中,ASHMI 也表现出多重疗效。因为在临床研究中 ASHMI 提高了 IFN-γ 水平,并使皮质醇水平正常化,所以进一步的临床试验应确定当 ASHMI 与皮质类固醇联合使用时,是否能修复/规范 IFN-γ 和皮质醇水平。识别 ASHMI 中活性化合物将加强我们对其药理学机制的理解,并可能发现哮喘治疗的新药物。

(在研究中,ASHMI 不是唯一的以作为中药来源的哮喘治疗方法。在以上引用的评论文章中可找到更加完整的讨论。)

李秀敏博士已在其诊所中使用 ASHMI,在那里它被用作补充剂而不是药物。她说:"我们必须要小心。我们的湿疹治疗从第一天开始就是用的类固醇,你不能突然停药并转用一些新的药物,因为当新的治疗方法生效时,炎症可能复发。我们会引进新的疗法并逐渐减少类固醇。自始至终,我们记录着 IgE 水平和肺功能,

① Min-Li H, Ying S, Xiu-Min L. Effects and mechanisms of actions of Chinese herbal medicines for asthma[J]. Chinese Journal of Integrative Medicine, 2011, 17(7): 483-491.

② Ibid. p. 485.

seeing in our clinical trials. That is, ASHMI has clinical efficacy. ”

Cancer

No discussion of the capacity of herbal medicine to modulate the immune system (or excite the world about the possibilities) would be complete without including cancer. In 1971, President Richard Nixon signed the National Cancer Act, also known as the "War on Cancer. " Trillions of dollars have been spent to fund basic research on the molecular mechanisms behind cell division and their regulation. Trillions more have been spent on treatments, but cancer remains a tremendous drain on patient health and finances. As I am writing this, The *New York Times* (April 24, 2013) carries a story "Doctors Denounce Cancer Drug Prices of $ 100,000 a Year", which explains that "more than 100 influential cancer specialists from around the world have taken the unusual step of banding together in hopes of persuading some leading pharmaceutical companies to bring prices down. "

Maybe it didn't have to be this way. There was a point more than a century ago when the industrial model of cancer treatment was paralleled by research on the immune system. In 2012, Dr. Jerome Groopman published an article in *The New Yorker* called "The T-Cell Army,"[①] which tells the story of a New York surgeon named William Coley who lost a patient, Elizabeth Dashiell, to sarcoma in 1891 and devoted himself to finding a cure. In the records of New York Hospital, He found one patient who stood out from the grim stories. Eleven years earlier, Fred Stein, a German immigrant who worked as a housepainter, had

---

① http://www. newyorker. com/reporting/2012/04/23/12042 3 fa_fact_groopman#ixzz2NcyoxyDC.

这证实了我们在临床试验中看到的,即 ASHMI 具有临床疗效。"

癌症

如果不包括癌症,任何关于草药调节免疫系统的能力(或激发世界对其可能性的讨论)的讨论都是不完整的。1971 年,理查德·尼克松总统签署了《国家癌症法案》,也被称为"向癌症宣战"。数万亿美元花费在细胞分裂和其调节后的有关分子机制的基础研究中。更多的数万亿花费在治疗上,但癌症仍然是对患者健康和财务的巨大消耗。当我写这篇文章时,《纽约时报》(2013 年 4 月 24 日)刊登了一篇《医生谴责每年 10 万美元的癌症药物价格》的报道,这篇文章解释"超过 100 位来自世界各地有影响力的癌症专家已采取了不同寻常的联合步骤,并希望说服一些主要的制药公司降低价格。"

也许没必要这样做。一个多世纪以前,癌症治疗的工业模式与免疫系统的研究并驾齐驱。在 2012 年,杰罗姆·古罗柏曼博士在《纽约客》杂志发表了一篇名为《T 细胞大军》的文章,讲述了 1891 年纽约外科医生威廉·科利的患者伊丽莎白·达希尔因恶性毒瘤离世,他致力于找到一种治疗方法的故事。威廉·科利从纽约医院的记录中发现一名突出的患者。11 年前,房屋油漆工德国移民弗瑞德·斯坦,其颈部出现一颗

a rapidly growing sarcoma in his neck. After four operations and four recurrences of the cancer, a senior surgeon declared Stein's case "absolutely hopeless." Then an infection caused by streptococcal bacteria broke out in red patches across Stein's neck and face. There were no antibiotics at the time, so his immune system was left to fight off the infection unaided. Remarkably, as his white blood cells combatted the bacteria, the sarcoma shrank into a bland scar. Stein left the hospital with no infection and no discernible cancer. Coley concluded that something in Stein's own body had shrunk the cancer.

Groopman tells us that for a decade, Coley pursued the hypothesis that the immune system could be harnessed for cancer, which one colleague called "whispers of nature," supported by John D. Rockefeller, who had been personally close to the deceased Miss Dashiell. At the same time, Rockefeller was backing the work of Dr. James Ewing, who thought that the newly discovered miracle of radiation was the only treatment for cancer. The Rockefeller family's interest in cancer treatment had begun with John D. 's father, "Doctor William A. Rockefeller, the Celebrated Cancer Specialist," who sold a treatment made of—what else? —the crude oil that provided the basis for the family fortune. ①

Eventually, Rockefeller threw his money behind the industrial model that led to our current reliance on radiation and chemotherapy, whose side effects are so dire that they sound like the medical version of the Vietnam War pronouncement "We had to destroy the

快速增长的恶性毒瘤。在四次手术和四次复发后,一名资深外科医生声称斯坦的病情"毫无希望"。然后,由链球菌引起的感染在斯坦的脖子和脸上爆发出红色斑块。在那时没有抗生素,因此他的免疫系统独自对抗感染。值得注意的是,因为他的白细胞与细菌斗争,所以恶性毒瘤萎缩成一个淡淡的疤痕。斯坦离开了医院,毫无感染且无明显癌症。科利推断斯坦体内的某种物质可治愈癌症。

古罗柏曼告诉我们,在十年的时间里,科利一直致力于证实免疫系统可被激发以治疗癌症的假设,一位同事称之为"大自然的低语",与已故达希尔女士关系密切的约翰·D. 洛克菲勒也对此提供支持。同时,洛克菲勒支持了詹姆斯·尤因博士的工作。詹姆斯·尤因博士认为新发现的放疗奇迹是治疗癌症的唯一方法。洛克菲勒家族对癌症治疗的兴趣开始于约翰·D. 的父亲威廉·A. 洛克菲勒博士,著名的癌症专家。他出售了一种由某东西构成的疗法——还有什么?——为家族财富提供基础的原油。

最后,洛克菲勒把钱投给了导致我们目前依赖放射和化疗的工业化癌症治疗模式,其副作用也是可怕的,它们听起来就像是越南战争声明的医疗版本"为了拯救它,我们不得

---

① Ron R. Tales from the cancer cure underground[M]// The Secret Parts of Fortune. New York: Random House, 2000.

village in order to save it. "

Now, however, there is a resurgence of interest in exploring the possibility of using the immune system for cancer. In the months since Groopman's *New Yorker* piece came out, *The New York Times* has published several articles. One was about Dr. Ralph Steinman, who tried "to concoct a set of treatments from his body's own ingredients, which could take over from his chemotherapy and form a customized, dynamic treatment for his disease. "[①] Dr. Steinman died several hours before he was to be informed that he would be sharing a Nobel Prize, which put the award in doubt, because it's not to be given posthumously (an exception was made).

Another *Times* article was about the work of Dr. Suzanne L. Topalian, a melanoma specialist at Johns Hopkins University, on a drug to thwart a "molecular shield" that protects tumors from attacks by the immune system. [②]

A third tells of a young leukemia patient who was given a disabled HIV virus that reprogrammed her immune system to fight the cancer. [③]

Thus, we come to the potential of ASHMI for fighting cancer. A colleague of Dr. Li, Martin J. Walsh, PhD, Associate Professor of Structural and Chemical Biology, Pediatrics, Hepatology, and Genetics and Genomic Sciences, has investigated the

不摧毁村庄。"

然而,人们对探索使用免疫系统治疗癌症的可能性有了新的兴趣。古罗柏曼在《纽约客》的那篇文章发表后的几个月里,《纽约时报》已经发表了几篇文章。其中一篇是关于拉夫尔·斯坦曼博士,他试图"从人体自身成分中合成一种治疗方法,将代替化疗,并形成对自身疾病的特定的和动态的治疗方法。"斯坦曼博士去世后几小时被通知将分享诺贝尔奖,这使该奖项处于不确定之中,因为该奖项不可能授予去世的人(有一项例外)。

《纽约时报》的另一篇文章是关于约翰·霍普金斯大学的黑色素瘤专家苏珊娜·L.托帕利安博士的研究,研究一种可以融化"分子屏障"的药,这一屏障使得肿瘤免受免疫系统的攻击。

第三个故事讲述了一位年轻的白血病患者被注射了一种缺陷艾滋病病毒,该病毒重新编程了她的免疫系统以对抗癌症。

因此,我们发现了 ASHMI 对抗癌症的潜力。李秀敏博士的同事,马丁·J.沃尔什博士,结构和化学生物学、儿科、肝脏病学、遗传学和基因组科学副教授,与李秀敏博士在实验室

① http://www.nytimes.com/2012/12/23/ maga-zine/is-the-cure-for-cancer-inside-you.html.

② http://www.nytimes.com/2012/06/02/business/drug-helps-immune-system-fight-cancer.html? _r=0.

③ From the article "In Girl's Last Hope, Altered Immune Cells Beat Leukemia" in the *New York Times*.

possibilities in the laboratory in collaboration with Dr. Li. [1] He writes in the Abstract of an unpublished article called "Inhibition of Tumor Cell Growth by Herbal Preparation MSSM-03" :

The use of herbal medicine has been in use over several centuries with little known about either the biochemical basis or genetic mechanisms that regulate the actions of herbal medicine. Since the efficacy and safety profile of many herbal preparations have been unofficially validated, more government focus on the use of these medicinal products has allowed their use to be more widely accepted by the medical community at large with legal provisions for their use.

Because of the pleiotropic (producing more than one effect) actions of herbal medicine to direct broad activities over the host organism, it is likely that herbal medicines are comprised of several unknown bioreactive compounds that interact with several signaling pathways.

Walsh and his colleagues studied ASHMI—MSSM-03, which is its name for purposes of research at Mount Sinai School of Medicine—for its potential to suppress growth of tumor cells in culture. Using immunoblot analysis of tumor cells treated with MSSM-03, they found that after 18 hours, the proteins in tumor cells that inhibit growth increased, while those that encourage growth had separated into harmless components. They add, "These studies provide evidence that MSSM-03 is a tumor cell growth inhibitor and may indicate potential use in treatment of

里已研究了其可能性。他在名为《通过草药制剂 MSSM-03 抑制肿瘤细胞生长》的未发表文章的摘要中写道：

草药的使用已经有几个世纪的历史了，但人们对调节草药作用的生化基础或遗传机制知之甚少。由于许多草药制剂的有效性和安全性已经得到非官方的验证，政府对这些药物的使用更加重视，使得它们的使用得到医学界的广泛接受，并有了使用它们的法律规定。

由于草药具有多效性（产生一种以上效应）作用，从而引导宿主有机体上广泛的活动，草药很可能由几种未知的生物反应性化合物组成，这些化合物与几种信号通路相互作用。

沃尔什和其同事研究了 ASHMI——MSSM-03，这是它的名字，用于在西奈山医学院进行研究——因为它有可能抑制培养中肿瘤细胞的生长。使用免疫印迹法分析用 MSSM-03 处理的肿瘤细胞，他们发现 18 小时后，肿瘤细胞内抑制生长的蛋白质增加，而那些促进生长的蛋白质分成了无害的部分。他们又说："这些研究提供了证据，证明 MSSM-03 是肿瘤细胞生长抑制剂，并可能表明治疗增生性增长疾病例

---

[1] From the unpublished article "Inhibition of Tumor Cell Growth by Herbal Preparation MSSM-03".

hyperplastic growth diseases, such as cancer. "

⑮ Treating Severe Allergic Diseases: Three Cases from Private Clinical Practice

While Dr. Xiu-Min Li is an extraordinary scientist, she is also a great clinical practitioner, a healer. As Scott Sicherer says, in China, TCM is just medicine.

Dr. Li employs a much larger array of compounds at her private practice than are currently being studied. The medications qualify for use with patients as supplements with a long history of safe use and, as employed under Xiu-Min's standards, nontoxicity, although they are not reimbursable by insurance companies.

She introduced me to three families who have benefited from her treatments from among the dozens who have passed through her doors from states across this country, as well as from the United Kingdom, Spain, Canada, Australia, France, and India. Having spent the best part of this book explaining how these treatments work in theory, I also want you to see why Xiu-Min's faith in their efficacy is well founded, although these accounts qualify as anecdotal evidence, not scientifically verified. However Chinese doctors have arrived at their formulas and strategies over the centuries, those formulas and strategies do seem to work. I also wanted to share these stories because they point the way toward incorporating these treatments into Western clinical practice, Dr. Li's dream of integrative medicine.

Julie

Dr. Elena Simon (name changed) is an

如癌症的潜在用途。"

⑮ 治疗严重的过敏疾病:选自个人临床实践的三个案例

李秀敏博士是一名非凡的科学家,也是一名伟大的临床医生和治疗师。如斯科特·史可瑞所说,中医在中国就是医学。

李秀敏博士在她的私人诊所使用的混合物比目前研究的要多得多。依照李博士的标准所使用的药物,尽管它们在保险公司是不可报销的,但是这些药物有资格作为具有长期安全使用历史的补充剂用于患者。

来自美国各州,以及来自英国、西班牙、加拿大、澳大利亚、法国和印度的几十个家庭已经从她的治疗中受益,她给我介绍了其中的三个家庭。尽管这些描述可以作为轶事证据,而没有经过科学验证,但这本书的大部分内容解释这些疗法在理论上是怎么可行的,我还想让你们看到为什么李博士对其疗效的信念是有根据的。不管中医几个世纪以来如何制定出他们的配方和策略,这些配方和策略似乎确实奏效了。我也想分享这些故事,因为它们为将这些疗法融入西方临床实践指明了方向,这是李秀敏博士的中西医结合医学梦想。

朱莉

埃琳娜·西蒙博士(化名)是离

emergency room doctor at a community hospital two hours from Toronto who occasionally works shifts as long as 36 hours, depending on the availability of other doctors. She says that until the age of 14, her daughter Julie was an outgoing straight-A student and cheerleader with no health issues to speak of. One night three years ago, while out for dinner at a Thai restaurant with her father, Julie's life changed. She began to break out in hives, and her throat began to tighten. Her father took her to an emergency room— not the one where Elena works—where she was treated for anaphylaxis.

The local allergist tested Julie for allergies to peanut and tree nuts— staples of Thai cooking—but nothing stood out. Over the next several weeks, this scenario played out repeatedly, fortunately with three-hour delayed onset so there was sufficient time to react medically. With no adequate answers available in their rural community, the next stop was the Hospital for Sick Children in Toronto, (referred to by doctors as "Sick Kids"), where Elena had done part of her training in family medicine. Sick Kids has an allergy department, although there was no treatment in the hospital except to give epinephrine and antihistamines.

Julie became so reactive that she would react to trace allergens in her nut-free school. She couldn't walk through a grocery store without responding, and she ended up in the Toronto ER an average of every two weeks. After a lifetime as a star student, her repeated absences took a toll on her schoolwork. All told, Julie missed half a year of school over the next two years. "She spent so much time in the emergency room hooked up to IVs that she was on a first-name

多伦多有两小时路程的社区医院的急诊室医生,她偶尔轮班长达36小时,这取决于有没有其他医生可用。她说她的女儿朱莉14岁前一直是一名外向直率的优等生和啦啦队队长,毫无健康问题。但是,三年前的一个晚上,当朱莉和她的父亲在一家泰国餐馆吃晚饭的时候,朱莉的生活改变了。她开始突发荨麻疹,她的喉咙开始变紧。她的父亲立刻带她去急诊室(不是埃琳娜工作的地方),在那里她接受了过敏反应的治疗。

当地的过敏症专科医生检查了朱莉对花生和坚果(泰国菜的主要原料)的过敏反应,但是无明显情况发生。在接下来的几周,朱莉过敏的情景反复上演。幸运的是,发作具有三个小时的延迟,因此医学上有足够的时间进行对抗。在他们的所在农村社区没有充足的医疗资源,他们去了多伦多儿童医院(医生称为"患儿医院"),埃琳娜在那里接受了部分家庭医学培训。患儿有专门的过敏科室提供治疗,尽管医院除了给他们注射肾上腺素和抗组胺药物外,没有其他治疗方法。

朱莉变得如此敏感,以至于在她那所没有坚果的学校里,她都会对微量过敏原作出反应。她不可能在没有反应的情况下走过一家杂货店,平均每两周她就会出现在多伦多急诊室一次。在做了多年的优等生之后,她的反复缺课对她的学业产生了不良影响。总之,朱莉在接下来的两年里缺课达半年。"她花了太多时间在

basis with the entire staff. Whenever she returned, the ER nurses and doctors would say, ' You again. ' " Dr. Simon's own work began to suffer as well, as she was forced to deal with repeated emergencies and to provide homeschooling.

Elena told me, "Obviously, we couldn't go on like this. I began to suffer physically and emotionally, too. I'm a doctor, but I'm a mother first. But my problems were nothing compared to my daughter's. She became depressed for the first time in her life. She was put on prednisone and became moon-faced (a physical symptom of prolonged use of systemic steroids) and even suicidal. " A full-blown psychotic breakdown that required a late-night two-hour drive to Toronto was attributed to the prednisone, and the doctors took Julie off it. The head of psychiatry, a friend of Dr. Simon's at Sick Kids, said he had never seen anything like it. Removing the steroids improved Julie's state of mind but put her at greater risk of anaphylaxis.

The low point came when Julie went on an overnight camping trip on an island with her classmates, which is a traditional rite of passage for her school. Her mom gave her four EpiPens as well as antihistamines to take with her—and still, she had anaphylaxis. The helicopter ambulance couldn't land, so she had to be ferried to the opposite shore by canoe and put aboard an ambulance—at which point she had already used three EpiPens—all this in the middle of the night lighted by spotlights from the helicopter!

At last, Dr. Simon read about Dr. Li and FAHF-2. She made an appointment at Dr. Li's New York

急诊室静脉输液,以至于她和所有工作人员都是直呼其名。每次她到医院,急诊室的护士和医生都会说,'又是你。'"西蒙博士自己的工作也开始受到影响,因为她不得不处理反复出现的紧急情况,还要辅导功课。

埃琳娜告诉我:"显然,我们撑不住了。我的精神和情感也开始受到影响。我是一名医生,但首先我是一位母亲。但是我的问题不能和我女儿的问题相比。在她的生命中,她第一次感到沮丧。她使用泼尼松并且脸色苍白(长期使用全身性类固醇的身体症状),甚至有自杀倾向。"由于泼尼松导致的完全的精神崩溃,她深夜驾车两小时到多伦多,医生让朱莉停用泼尼松。精神科的主任,西蒙在多伦多儿童医院的朋友说他从未见过像这样的事情。停用类固醇改善了朱莉的精神状态,但使她面临更大的过敏风险。

低潮出现在朱莉和她的同学去一个岛上通宵野营旅行时,该旅行是她学校的传统的成人礼。虽然她的妈妈给了她四支肾上腺素笔和抗组胺药,但是她还是有过敏反应。直升机救护车不能着陆,因此不得不通过独木舟将她送到对岸,再放到救护车上。在此之前,她已经使用了三支肾上腺素笔。所有这一切都发生在直升机照明下的午夜时分!

最后,西蒙博士读到有关李秀敏博士和FAHF-2的事情。她预约了李

private clinic, where both mother and daughter acquired an instant sense of hope. "She was so warm and welcoming, and talked with us for two hours taking a full medical history. I believe in bedside manner, and I have never seen anything like this. She even gave Julie an acupuncture treatment."

Then began a regimen of 50 pills a day. Within 6 months, Julie had no hives at all and no constriction of her throat. Where she had been taking so much Benadryl that she was sleepy all the time, followed by a period in which it lost its sedating effects altogether, Julie has only taken two Benadryl in months for one minor reaction. She went back in school and graduated on time.

After a year on the treatment, life is now so normal that Julie is back to being a teenager, and impatient with the continued daily dosing, but Dr. Simon insists. "She has her life back. And Dr. Li is my medical hero."

Postscript from Dr. Simon: "Julie was just away in France taking a course this past month. Amazingly, she encountered nuts accidentally in a pastry and did not react. Then, she did not tell me but stopped taking the medicine while she was there and ate many nuts in pastries, including almonds, which she was very allergic to, and was fine! When she returned, she also ate a chocolate spread with mixed nuts in it in front of me, which she did not react to at all. She wants to continue without the medicine and see how things go. I almost cannot believe my eyes. She has been on the protocol for a year, taking it religiously."

秀敏博士在纽约的私人诊所,在这里母亲和女儿都立刻感觉获得了希望。"她是如此的温暖和热情,并与我们交谈了两小时,了解完整的病史。我相信医生对病人的态度,而且我从未见过这样的事情。她曾通过针灸给朱莉治疗。"

然后开始每天服用50片药。在6个月内,朱莉身上的荨麻疹全消失了,喉咙也无收紧感。因为她服用了太多的苯海拉明,所以她总是昏昏欲睡。在随后的一段时间里,该药失去了镇静效果,后来几个月里对于较小的反应,朱莉仅服用两片苯海拉明。她开始上学并且准时毕业了。

经过一年的治疗,朱莉现在的生活变得正常了,她又变成了正常的青少年,并且对每天持续服药感到不耐烦,但是西蒙博士仍然坚持。"她的生活恢复了。李秀敏博士是我的医学英雄。"

西蒙博士附言:"上个月,朱莉去法国学习。令人惊奇的是,她偶然吃了一个有坚果的糕点但是没有反应。她并没有告诉我,她停止了服药,然而她在法国又吃了很多有坚果的糕点,包括杏仁,这些都是她曾经过敏的,但是没事!当她回来后,她在我面前也吃了一些带有混合坚果的巧克力,她完全没有反应。她想要在不服药的情况下,继续尝试,看看情况如何。我几乎不能相信我的眼睛。她已经坚持这个医疗方案一年了,严格地坚持服药。"

Jackie

Jackie O. is a 10-year-old girl allergic to eggs, peanuts, fish, seeds, citrus fruits, and nuts, with a history of anaphylaxis, asthma, and total blood IgE of 6000. Although most allergists don't consider blood IgE levels as confirmation of food allergy on their own (history of reactivity is the surest sign), anything over 100 is considered high, and much lower levels do not preclude dangerous reactions. Levels as high as 6000 are indicative of serious allergies.

Although multiple food allergies were a big issue for Jackie, as they are for millions of others, the more immediate problem was that she suffered from severe intractable eczema. "It was everywhere," Jackie says, "my face, my neck, my eyelids, and down to my feet."

Her father, Greg, said to me, "It's terrible that an eight-year-old girl could be so self-conscious that she didn't want to go to school." Peer judgment aside, Jackie's teachers noticed her discomfort and were continually asking if she was all right.

She couldn't sleep through the night. "I used to wake up crying in the night. My friends thought I had polka-dot sheets because they had blood from scratching."

Says her father, "It was a big negative feedback loop. Lack of sleep weakened her immune system, leaving her vulnerable to other infections."

Jackie's allergist, who happened to be my cousin, Dr. Paul Ehrlich, tried all the conventional treatments: antihistamines, steroidal creams, and gauze wraps to

杰基

杰基·O. 是一个 10 岁的小女孩,她对鸡蛋、花生、鱼、种子、柑橘类水果和坚果过敏,并有过敏史、哮喘史和总血 IgE6 000 水平的病史。尽管许多过敏症专科医生不将血 IgE 水平视为食物过敏的证明(反应性历史是最可靠的标志),因为任何指标超过 100 都被认为是高的,而且低得多的水平并不排除危险的反应。高达 6 000 的水平表明严重过敏。

尽管多样食物过敏对杰基来说是一个大问题,就像其他数百万人一样,但更直接的问题是她患有严重的顽固性湿疹。杰基说:"湿疹到处都是,遍布我的脸、脖子、眼皮一直到我的脚。"

她的父亲格雷格对我说:"一个 8 岁的小女孩如此难为情,不想上学是很糟糕的事情。"先将同学的评论放一边,杰基的老师注意到她不舒服并不断询问她的身体状况。

她整晚都睡不着。"我过去常常在夜里哭着醒来。我的朋友们认为我有波点床单,因为床单染上了湿疹抓破后流的血。"

她父亲说:"这是一个巨大的负面反馈循环。缺乏睡眠削弱了她的免疫系统,使她容易受到其他感染。"

杰基的过敏症专科医生,恰巧是我的堂兄保罗·埃尔利希博士,他尝试了各种传统的疗法:抗组胺、类固醇乳

protect her skin from scratching fingers. "I looked like a mummy," says Jackie. Nothing worked. And then Paul did the New York equivalent of sending her to Lourdes. He referred her to Dr. Li's private clinic.

The first session consisted of a couple of hours of talk with Mom and Dad present, ending with Dr. Li's pronouncement, "I will try to help you." With the second session began a daily regimen of a special herbal soaking bath, and five kinds of capsules totaling 64 (which Jackie could not swallow so instead made them into a hot tea), and a nightly rub with a black cream called IABZC everywhere below the neck, waiting for five minutes before putting on her pajamas. Eventually she was able to swallow the capsules instead of making them into tea, and currently she is down to "just" 38 per day.

Within a month and a half, Jackie started to improve rapidly. "It was night and day," says her father. Jackie's teachers began to notice that the redness was going away and couldn't help commenting. Jackie's asthma was also better. After a bit more than two years of treatment, Jackie's skin is so normal that she has to be reminded as she's going out the door for school in the morning to take her pills, which she finds as disgusting as the tea, and she faces two to three more years of treatment.

Paul follows up on Jackie's IgE levels and her liver and kidney function annually. Her total IgE went down from ～6000 to ～3000 after one year of treatment and to ～1800 after two years of treatment. Peanut IgE reduced about tenfold (from ～30 to 3); tree nut, fish, and sesame IgE levels also went down. Jackie's liver

霜和纱布包裹,以保护她的皮肤免受手指抓伤。杰基说:"我看起来像木乃伊。"但毫无效果。之后,保罗在纽约所做的相当于把她送去卢尔德。他向她推荐了李秀敏博士的私人诊所。

第一次见面包括父母在场的情况下进行几个小时的交谈,最后李医生说:"我会尽力帮助你们。"第二次见面,每日一次的特殊的草药泡浴开始了,还有五种胶囊总计64粒(杰基吞不下,所以把它们泡进热水),并在晚上用一种名为IABZC的黑色药膏在颈部以下的各处按摩,等待五分钟后才穿她的睡衣。最终,她能够吞下胶囊,而不用把它们制成茶,现在她每天"只"吃38粒胶囊。

不到一个半月,杰基就开始快速恢复。"简直就是天壤之别,"她父亲说。她的老师们也开始注意到她的皮肤红肿在消退并且忍不住议论。而且她的哮喘也好转了。经过两年多一点的治疗以后,杰基的皮肤恢复得很正常了,以至于不得不有人提醒她出门上学前要吃药,虽然她觉得吃药就像喝茶一样讨厌,但她还要接受两到三年的治疗。

保罗每年都追踪记录杰基的IgE水平和肝肾功能。一年后,她的总IgE从6 000下降到3 000,经过两年的治疗后,下降到了1 800。花生IgE降低了大约10倍(从30到3);坚果、鱼和芝麻IgE水平也下降了。

and kidney function are all in normal range.

Her father says, "How can these ingredients I can't pronounce make her so much better?"

Jackie can pronounce the name of Dr. Li's herbal medicines. She gave Dr. Li a gift, which is a drawing in Chinese characters meaning "harmony" and "hope." Jackie says of Dr. Li, "She changed my life. Without her, I wouldn't be sitting here with a smile on my face."

The story gets better. After a few months of treatment, Dr. Li approved more strenuous aerobic activity to strengthen Jackie's lungs. Jackie has been riding a two-wheeler since she was four with her dad every chance she got and at age nine joined the children's cycling team Star Track in NYC. After a year of treatment, her asthma had improved so much that she won several local races as well as the New York State Championship for her age division. This gave her enough confidence to set a goal for the 2013 Junior National Championships. In July of 2013, as the second youngest competitor in the girl's 10 – 12 division, she finished 17th in the time trial and 15th in the road race and promptly crowned herself "fastest 10-year-old female cyclist in the US." "It was such a major victory for her just to be there," her dad said. "To think where she was two and a half years ago, and now she is competing against the best girls her age in the country is nothing short of a miracle."

▌Aaron

Aaron (name changed) was a colicky baby. As he began eating solids at the age of six months, he started projectile vomiting frequently, but without

而她的肝肾功能也都在正常范围内。

她的父亲说:"这些我叫不出名的成分是如何使她变好的?"

杰基知道李秀敏博士的草药的名字。她送给李秀敏博士一份礼物——用汉字写的意为"和谐"和"希望"的画。杰基谈到李秀敏博士时说:"她改变了我的生活。没有她,我不能满面笑容地坐在这里。"

治疗很顺利。几个月的治疗后,李秀敏博士同意进行更多剧烈的有氧运动以增强杰基的肺功能。杰基四岁后只要一有机会就和她的父亲一起骑自行车,九岁时加入纽约的Star Track 儿童自行车队。经过一年的治疗,她的哮喘改善了很多,因此她赢得了几个当地比赛以及自己年龄组的纽约州锦标赛总冠军。这给了她足够的自信确立2013青少年全国总冠军的目标。在2013年7月,作为10~12岁女子组的第二小的选手,她拿到了计时赛第17,越野赛第15的成绩,并且立即被冠以"美国最快的10岁女子自行车手"。她的爸爸说:"对于她来说,站在那里是多大的胜利啊!想想她两年半前的处境,而现在她与全国同龄人中的佼佼者竞争,这简直是个奇迹。"

▌亚伦

亚伦(化名)是一个患有腹痛的婴儿。自从他六个月大开始吃固体食物时,他开始频繁地喷射性呕吐,

pattern. The pediatrician recommended scaling back his diet to breast milk and rice cereal. Foods were reintroduced and new foods were introduced without any problems for a few weeks. The cycle soon would soon begin again, however, so Aaron's parents would scale back to the basics, then reintroduce other food, and again, the roller coaster would start. The pediatrician didn't have any answers.

Kate, Aaron's mother, took the 10-month-old boy to see a pediatric gastroenterologist who suggested that the problem might be celiac disease (an immune reaction to gluten, a protein in wheat, barley, and rye) or possibly food allergies. The doctor tested Aaron, who had 3 of the 4 markers for celiac, and wanted to "scope" him (pass an endoscope through his mouth and stomach to take a tissue sample from his small intestine). Anxious to spare their son the trauma, however, Aaron's parents took him for a second opinion at Miami Children's Hospital, where the GI specialist recommended against it.

Aaron was also referred to an allergist who conducted RASTs, which showed sensitivity to eight foods. The allergist told Kate to keep all of these foods out of the boy's diet, despite the fact that on many days, he would eat the foods and not have any allergic reaction. Kate tried the elimination diet. Aaron experienced hives at 12 months after consuming dairy and at 15 months after consuming baked egg whites.

The vomiting cycle continued. When Aaron was 12 months old, the pediatrician prescribed Zantac, an

但没有规律。儿科医生建议他减少饮食,只吃母乳和米粉。他父母为他重新制定了食谱,新食谱在开始几周几不会引发过敏。但是,很快他又开始呕吐,然后又重新制定食谱,这种循环每隔一段时间就会出现,他的父母只得又回到基本食谱,很快,循环会再次出现。儿科医生也束手无策。

10 个月大时,亚伦的母亲凯特带着他去看儿科胃肠病医生,医生诊断可能是乳糜泻(一种对谷蛋白的免疫反应,谷蛋白是小麦、大麦和黑麦里的一种蛋白质),或可能是食物过敏。医生检测出亚伦具有 4 个乳糜泻腹腔标记物中的 3 个,并且想给他做镜检(从嘴插入内窥镜,经过胃到达小肠取组织样本)。虽然急于让儿子从疾病中解脱,但亚伦的父母采取了第二个意见,并带他去迈阿密儿童医院进行检查,在这里肠胃专家建议不做检查。

亚伦也被推荐给做放射过敏原吸附试验的过敏症专科医生,结果显示他对八种食物过敏。过敏症专科医生告诉凯特将所有这些食物从他的饮食中去除,尽管如此,很多次即使亚伦吃了这些食物但却没有任何过敏反应。凯特尝试排除饮食。但亚伦还是得了两次荨麻疹,一次是他 12 个月大的时候,因为喝了牛奶,还有一次是他 15 个月大的时候,因为吃了煎蛋清。

呕吐循环还在继续。亚伦 12 个月大的时候,儿科医生给他开了一种

anti-reflux medicine, for a year, which seemed to help as the vomiting episodes subsided.

Eating at restaurants wasn't much of a problem because there were many restaurants that were kosher for either meat or dairy. As Aaron's family learned, however, there is a difference between *parve*—dairy free for religious purposes, which is determined by weight—and completely dairy *protein*-free. Still, kosher restaurants that served meat did provide some leeway. Even this was not enough, however, when two-year-old Aaron began playing with hummus that was served instead of butter with bread on the tables and reacted to the sesame it contained. Other foods provoked hives, facial swelling, and vomiting.

Aaron's food and environmental allergen list grew, and more things were dropped from his diet. The doctors projected that he might outgrow his allergies by age 3, then 5, then 8, and 10. Aaron had trouble gaining weight and growing. He came home early from school regularly because of allergic reactions to food in science experiments and in special treats. Aaron's throat became itchy just being near the popcorn popped in the school courtyard as a Friday-afternoon treat. Kate added accommodations to Aaron's "504 plan," which refers to Section 504 of the Rehabilitation Act and the Americans with Disabilities Act, specifying that no one with a disability can be excluded from participating in federally funded programs or activities at school. No science experiment dealing with food could include any of his allergens; a week's notice of any activities

治疗胃酸倒流的药善胃得,在开始的一年里善胃得似乎是有效的,因为呕吐发生得少了。

因为许多餐馆的肉或奶制品经过犹太洁食认证,所以在餐馆吃饭也不是大问题。然而,正如亚伦的家人所了解到的那样,具有宗教意义的无乳制品是由体重决定的,这和完全不含蛋白质的乳制品不同。但是,提供肉类的犹太洁食餐馆确实提供了一些余地。但情况还是不太理想,当两岁的亚伦吃了餐桌上提供的鹰嘴豆泥而不是黄油搭配的面包时,其所含的成分芝麻让他起了反应,而其他食物也同样让他出现荨麻疹、面部红肿和呕吐现象。

随着致敏食物和环境过敏原不断增多,亚伦的饮食中减少了更多东西。医生们预测,他可能会在3岁时变得不再过敏,然后又说5岁,8岁,10岁。亚伦很难增重或长高。因为对科学实验和特色餐中的食物过敏,他经常提早放学回家。每周五下午学校都会在院子里做爆米花来款待孩子们,但亚伦只要接近爆米花,他的喉咙就会发痒。凯特在亚伦的"504计划"中添加了食宿,"504计划"指的是《康复法》和《美国残疾人法》的第504节,规定任何残疾人都不能被排除在参加联邦资助的项目或学校活动之外。有关食物的任何科学实验都不能包括亚伦的任何过敏原;任何涉及食物的活动都必须提前一周通知凯特,这样她才能保护她

involving food must be given to Kate so she could help protect her son.

Allergy shots were initiated for Aaron's environmental allergens, but the big problem was eating. At 9 years old, he was having problems again with intermittent vomiting and diarrhea, except it was worse this time. He couldn't keep food or liquid down, and after each vomiting episode, he remained lethargic for a day or two. After a trip to the ER for dehydration (and during which he could not take the hospital's anti-vomiting medication because the inactive ingredients included an allergen), he saw another gastroenterologist.

Eventually, Aaron was diagnosed with EoE, an allergic condition mediated not by mast cells but other effector cells called eosinophils that show up where they don't belong. These reactions can be delayed 12 to 48 hours after exposure to an allergen, possibly, as new research shows,[①] because they are triggered by basophils, the effector cells associated with late-phase IgE-mediated allergies. Day-to-day existence became, in Kate's words, "a fine line between quality of life and sustenance." The wrong foods would result in hours of vomiting and diarrhea, followed by 24 - 48 hours of lethargy. At age 11, Aaron weighed just 59 pounds.

Disappointed by conventional treatment, Kate began researching alternatives, including OIT and FAHF-2 trials, but EoE was disqualifying for all those. However, Kate brought Aaron to see Dr. Li in her

的儿子。

亚伦开始接受过敏疫苗注射来治疗环境过敏原问题,但是最大的问题是饮食。在 9 岁的时候,他又出现了间歇性呕吐和腹泻,但这次情况更糟。他无法咽下食物或者液体。每次呕吐复发后,他就会昏昏欲睡一两天,因为脱水他被送入急诊室后(在此期间,由于非活性成分包含过敏原,他不能摄入医院的抗呕吐药物),他接受了另一个胃肠病医生的治疗。

最终,亚伦被诊断患有嗜酸性粒细胞性食管炎,一种不是由肥大细胞引起的过敏性疾病,而是由其他被称为嗜酸性粒细胞的效应细胞出现在不该出现的地方引起的。新研究表明,因为它们由嗜碱性粒细胞触发,嗜碱性粒细胞是与晚期 IgE 介导的过敏相关的效应细胞,所以接触过敏原后,这些反应很可能延迟 12 至 48 个小时。用凯特的话来说,日常生活的状况是,"生活质量和生存之间只有一线之隔"。食用不当的食物就会导致几小时的呕吐和腹泻,接下来是 24 ~ 48 小时的嗜睡。11 岁的亚伦体重仅为59 磅。

对常规治疗感到失望后,凯特开始研究替代疗法,包括 OIT 和 FAHF-2 试验,但是这些对于嗜酸性粒细胞性食管炎均不适用。然而,当凯特将亚伦带

---

① http：//www. nature. com/nm/journal/vl9/n8/full/nm. 3281. html.

private clinic, where he received a regimen of herbal medications to reduce his eosinophils and allergic reactions. The medication regimen includes *Mei Huang Tea* III pills, Digestive Tea capsules, *Huo Xiang Zheng Qi Wan* pills, Seasonal Herbal capsules, bath additives, and skin creams. After 6 months, Aaron was asymptomatic and his eczema had improved.

A year after treatment commenced, the differences in Aaron's health and quality of life were "night and day," according to his mother. He gained weight. His breathing was much better, particularly at night. His eosinophil count, although still high at 69, was down from 225. Aaron's reactions grew milder and milder. A reaction on January 8, 2013, at 8:30 am—thought to be a delayed reaction—was so mild that he was in school at 11:30. He had no other reactions until June when he reacted 36 hours after a baked egg challenge. In July, he passed a pecan challenge. Outside the immediate family, the person most deeply impressed by Aaron's improvement was the school nurse. Her job was much less frantic in the last six months of the school year because Aaron was no longer a frequent visitor.

16 The Slow Road to Clinical Practice

The earliest publications of Dr. Li's research that have led to the clinical trials now underway are almost 20 years old, with more years of research still to come. The journey to clinical practice is not just a matter of research, however. There are also matters of culture and custom, both for patients and for doctors.

Will people accept these therapies? Judging by the numbers of patients who have sought CAM treatments

到李秀敏博士的私人诊所时,他接受了一种草药疗法来减少他的嗜酸性粒细胞和过敏反应。药物治疗方案包括梅黄茶三剂、消化性茶胶囊、藿香正气丸片、四季草胶囊、沐浴添加剂以及护肤霜。6个月后,亚伦没有出现过敏症状并且他的湿疹也改善了。

经过一年的治疗以后,他的妈妈说:亚伦的健康和生活质量发生了天翻地覆的变化。他的体重增加了,他的呼吸状况更好了,尤其是晚上的时候。尽管他的嗜酸性粒细胞指数仍然很高,但是从225降到了69。亚伦的过敏反应越来越轻微。2013年1月8日上午8:30,他出现了反应,因为应该是延迟反应,反应很轻微,他11:30到学校了。期间没有其他反应,直到6月,他在煎蛋刺激36小时后才出现反应。7月,他通过了山核桃刺激。除了直系亲属以外,对亚伦的恢复印象最为深刻的应该就是学校护士了。她的工作在学年的最后六个月不再那么紧张,因为亚伦不是常客了。

16 缓慢的临床实践之路

李秀敏博士的研究成果最早发表于20年前,目前正在进行临床试验,未来还会有更多的研究。然而,通往临床实践的旅程不仅仅是一个研究问题。对病人和医生来说,还有文化和习俗的问题。

人们会接受这些治疗方法吗?从寻求补充和替代医学治疗(见第1

(see chapter 1), the demand side is already there. Anxious parents are clearly clamoring for results. This is why, after all, what we might call an OIT underground has sprung up, not to mention many treatments that have their origins in what we might call the web-footed school of medicine.

The question then becomes who will provide these treatments. Will physicians adopt new medications that come from outside the pharmaceutical mainstream? Dr. Lisa Sanders has written, "Doctors are not known for their rapid embrace of the new ... Physicians are so reluctant to change the way they practice medicine that it takes an average seventeen years for techniques well established by research—such as giving an aspirin to a patient having a heart attack—to be adopted by even half of those in practice."① In his book *How Doctors Think*, Dr. Jerome Groopman cites Douglas Watson, former president and CEO of Novartis, to the effect that research shows that most physicians regularly prescribe around two dozen drugs, most of which they learned about during their training, although their training may have taken place many years earlier.② I have no reason to think it's any different with allergists. *③

篇）的患者数量进行判定，需求方已经存在。焦急的父母强烈要求看到治疗成果。因此，这就是我们可以称为地下组织的 OIT 已经兴起的原因，更不用说那些我们称之为发源于三流医学院的许多疗法。

接下来的问题变成了谁将提供这些疗法。医生是否会采用主流药以外的新药物？丽莎·桑德斯博士写道："医生们不能快速接受新药物……医生们不愿意改变他们行医的方式。经过研究而确定的医疗技术，比如给心脏病发作的患者服用阿司匹林，平均需要 17 年的时间才能被一半的实践者采用。"在《医生如何思考》中，杰罗姆·古罗柏曼博士引用诺华公司前总裁兼首席执行官道格拉斯·沃森的话：研究表明，大多数医生经常开大约 24 种药物，其中大部分是他们在培训期间学到的，尽管他们的培训可能早已过去很多年。我没有理由认为（他们）与过敏症医生有任何不同。

---

① Lisa S. Every patient tells a story[M]. New York: Broadway Books, 2009.

② Groopman, op cit. p. 219.

③ *The one potentially game-changing tool I am familiar with is component testing, which helps establish which components of allergenic proteins a person reacts to, and can help predict the severity of allergic reactions, although it is nowhere near definitive. Years after component testing's FDA approval, many allergists continue to rely on testing technology that is widely acknowledged to be obsolete. (I must point out that I was paid by the manufacturer, ThermoFisherScientific *all too briefly* several years go to supply news items for its consumer blog. I continue to talk with the company's personnel regularly because they still represent the cutting edge in testing.)

我熟悉的一个可能改变游戏规则的工具是成分测试，它可以帮助确定一个人对过敏性蛋白的哪些成分作出反应，并且可以帮助预测过敏反应的严重程度，尽管它远不是决定性的。FDA 批准成分检测后几年内，许多过敏症专科医师继续依赖普遍认为是过时的检测技术。（我必须指出，几年来，由制造商赛默飞世尔科技公司支付以便向消费者提供新项目。我定期与公司人员交谈，因为他们仍然代表测试技术的最前沿。）

Dr. Renata Engler of Walter Reed National Military Medical Center is one of Dr. Li's greatest admirers. She described the dimensions of the challenge in a 2000 article about Dr. Li's early research:

The scope of what is included in the array of CAM treatments can be overwhelming to the health care providers trying to learn about them. Herbal medicine alone encompasses several textbooks of information but with no well-defined "evidence-based" guidelines or easily accessed educational material. Most physicians complain of difficulty remaining current with the knowledge required for the practice of allopathic medicine. Therapeutic arenas such as herbal medicine (with more than 1,800 herbals currently available on the US market) are overwhelming in informational content. It has been easier to ignore the whole area of CAM as "placebo" or "not effective" and many patients complain that it is difficult to find a health care provider willing to partner with alternative practitioners or to monitor them if they choose an herbal or other CAM therapeutic trial outside the Food and Drug Administration-approved pharmaceutical industry." (p. 628)

Thirteen years later, Dr. Engler remains skeptical about mainstream allergy practice meeting patient needs, and about practitioners' receptivity to CAM. She told me, "The system is currently failing a lot of patients. There's a tendency to abandon those who don't fit into comfortable evidence-based slots. This includes a high percentage of asthma cases and food-allergy patients. Our community consigns patients to hopelessness or treatments that are worse than the

沃尔特里德国家军事医疗中心的勒娜特·恩格勒博士是李秀敏博士崇拜者之一。2000 年的一篇关于李秀敏博士早期研究的文章描述了此项挑战的维度:

CAM 疗法的数列中包含的范围对试图了解它们的医疗保健提供者来说已经超出他们现今能够接受的范围。仅草药就包含了几本教科书的信息,但没有明确"基于证据"的指导方针或易于获取的教育材料。大多数医生抱怨说,他们很难掌握对抗疗法所需的知识。像草药(在美国市场上有超过 1800 种草药)的治疗领域在信息和内容方面让他们应接不暇。作为"安慰剂"或"无效果",我们更容易忽视整个 CAM 领域。许多患者抱怨说,很难找到愿意与其他医生合作的医疗保健提供者,或者当患者选择了在食品和药品管理局批准的医药行业之外的草药或其他的治疗试验时监督他们。(第628 页)

13 年后,恩格勒博士仍然对主流的过敏治疗方法能否满足病人的需要,以及医生对 CAM 的接受性持怀疑态度。她告诉我:"目前,该系统使大多数患者大失所望。现在有一个趋势,即放弃那些使用不符合循证医学疗法的患者。这包括高比例哮喘病例和食物过敏患者。医学界现在使患者感到绝望或是让患者接

disease. Steroids haven't answered the mail for everyone. "

Engler also blames the high-altitude perspective of certain regulators who control the financial spigot, citing a colleague whose funding was turned off because the decision makers were no longer interested in "individual patients." Her critique extends to the national research agenda: "Fifty percent of evidence-based medicine is significantly revised and/or reversed in five years. Most money goes into confirming what we already know instead of focusing on the gaps where we could add information."

However, other regulators show signs of a more expansive attitude toward alternatives. Acupuncture needles have been recognized as medical devices, and health insurance often covers part of the cost of treatment. Dr. Li says, " Current methodology of clinical trials does not totally fit the nature of traditional Chinese medicine, which is a more personalized medicine. The NIH encourages investigators to develop a more sophisticated methodology for clinical studies of complementary and alternative medicines. "

According to Dr. Li, FAHF-2 faces 8 to 10 more years of clinical trials (and tens of millions of dollars) before it will qualify as a pharmaceutical that can be reimbursable under current FDA standards and prescribed by practicing allergists with no special training. She says, "The FDA has issued guidance for botanical drug investigation. Some herbal medicines may be classified as prescription drugs after completing the clinical trials. " The current state of regulation with Dr. Li's unique circumstances does offer an

受比疾病本身更糟糕的治疗。类固醇不会治愈每一个人。"

恩格勒还指责某些控制金融龙头的监管机构的上帝视角,引用一位资金被切断的同事的故事,因为决策者不再对"个别病人"感兴趣。她的批评延伸到国家研究议程:"五年内,50%的循证医学应该得到显著修订和/或逆转。现在大多数钱都花在确认我们已经知道的事情上,而不关注我们可以补充的空白。"

然而,其他监管机构显示出对替代方案更宽松态度的迹象。针灸针被视为医疗器械,并且健康保险经常包含部分治疗费用。李秀敏博士说:"当前临床试验方法并不完全符合中医的本质,中医是更个性化的治疗。NIH鼓励研究人员为补充和替代药物的临床研究开发一种更成熟的方法。"

根据李秀敏博士的研究,FAHF-2要经过8到10年的临床试验(还要花费数千万美元)之后才有资格成为一种药物,可以根据现行的FDA标准得以报销,并由不经过特殊培训的过敏学家开出药方。她说:"FDA已经发布了植物药物试验的指南。完成临床试验后,一些草药可归类为处方药。"然而,由于李秀敏博士独特的情况,当前的监管状态确实提供了治疗的过渡路径。

intermediate road to treatment, however.

For one thing, some traditional Chinese medicines are already cleared for use as "dietary supplements." For another, they have a track record. Traditional Chinese medicines are regulated as medicines in China, Japan, and Korea, where they are part of mainstream medical care, are prescribed by doctors, and are dispensed in hospital pharmacies. They can also be used as over-the-counter medicines. Australia has also endorsed the use of some classical medicines based on a long history of safe and effective use. Finally, the medicines that Dr. Li uses already pass the most rigorous standards for safety and purity in the world, based on their certification both in China and at the lab at Mount Sinai.

Given the ineffectiveness of current practice at treating food allergies, I have a feeling that if there were a food-allergy pill today, many allergists would prescribe it, if only because they have so few options. Some doctors are openly frustrated at the limitations of today's medicine. I heard Dr. John Oppenheimer of New Jersey, who has had a distinguished career in both allergy research and practice, lament the fact that he often felt more like a risk manager than a healer.

Dr. Anna Nowak-Wegzryn, Dr. Li's colleague at Mount Sinai, told me that the fact that FAHF-2 is botanical in origin and has the aura of alternative medicine around it wouldn't be an impediment: "We use botanical-based drugs all the time." Surveys also show that, all things being equal, patients and their parents would prefer "natural" remedies to synthetic ones.

一方面,一些传统中药已经被批准作为"膳食补充剂"使用。另一方面,他们具有可追踪的记录。在中国、日本和韩国,传统中药是主流医疗保健的一部分并受到监管,由医生开处方,并在医院药房里配药。他们也可以用作非处方药。澳大利亚也赞同在长期安全和有效使用的基础上使用一些传统药物。最终,在中国和西奈山实验室的认证基础上,李秀敏博士使用的药物已经通过世界上最严格的安全和纯度标准(认证)。

鉴于当前医学在治疗食物过敏方面的效果不佳,我认为如果现今有一种治疗食物过敏的药物,许多过敏症专科医师就会因为选择太少而为病人开这种药。一些医生对当今的药物局限性感到沮丧。我听说来自新泽西州的约翰·奥本海默博士,在过敏研究和实践中都有杰出的贡献,哀叹他经常感觉自己更像一个风险管理者而不是一个治疗者。

李秀敏博士在西奈山医院的同事安娜·诺瓦卡-威格森博士告诉我这个事实:FAHF-2 本质上是植物药,头顶替代医学的"光环"对其不是障碍。"我们一直在使用植物性药物。"调查也显示,在所有条件相同的情况下,比起合成疗法,患者和其父母更喜欢"自然"疗法。

Certainly, I don't expect that allergists, even newly minted ones, will achieve grounding in alternative and complementary medicine any time soon. Allergy fellows (and there aren't a lot of them) learn from older doctors (few of whom, if any, have the necessary background).

Dr. Engler and several colleagues described the challenge of acquiring the necessary expertise in their aptly named article "Complementary and Alternative Medicine for the Allergist-Immunologist: Where Do I Start?"[①]

They say, Allergy-immunology specialists are faced with the challenge of how to respond practically to the evolving information presented by the expanding world of CAM. The spectrum of positions on CAM within conventional medical practices ranges from "don't ask, don't tell" to establishing a partnership with the patient who may be seeking or is already using CAM therapies. A small percentage of practitioners are incorporating both conventional and nontraditional medical therapies, reflecting a movement toward integrative medicine. Many physicians and health care workers in general are interested in learning more about CAM but are overwhelmed by the amount of information and afraid of entering into any discussions with their patients because of a possible liability risk and/or time requirement.

Furthermore, Dr. Engler and her coauthors point out that the magnitude of new information to assimilate on top of what they already know is daunting:

当然，我不指望过敏症专科医师，甚至是新晋医生，很快就能掌握替代和补充医学中的基础知识。过敏研究员（没有很多人）向资深医生学习（如有，很少的医生具有必要的医学背景）。

恩格勒博士和几位同事《过敏反应免疫学家的补充和替代医学：我该从哪里开始？》一文中描述了获得必要专业知识的挑战，这篇文章的标题切中要害。

他们说过敏免疫学专家面临的挑战是如何应对不断扩大的 CAM 世界所呈现的不断发展的信息。在常规医学实践中，CAM 的位置范围从"不问，不说"到与可能正在寻求或已经在使用 CAM 疗法的患者建立伙伴关系。一小部分的执业医师结合了常规和非常规药物治疗，反映出一种向综合医学的转变。一般来说，许多内科医生和健康护理工作者有兴趣学习更多关于 CAM 的知识，但由于信息太多，而且可能存在责任风险和/或时间要求，他们害怕与患者进行讨论。

此外，恩格勒博士和她的合著者指出，在他们已知的基础上需要接受大量的新信息，这令人生畏：

---

① Engler, et al., op cit.

The key elements of physician-patient interactions that involve CAM questions and/or therapeutic impact include the following: (1) exploring factors driving interest in CAM; (2) documenting clinical reasons for seeking CAM options; (3) assessing current disease/health status and therapies to date; (4) documenting patient's preferences and reasons; (5) assessing and documenting adequacy of medical evaluation; (6) defining a plan for follow-up visits; (7) providing good risk communications with option for additional consultative visits; (8) acknowledging evolving expectations and goals; (9) educating about new safety and/or efficacy issues related to CAM choices during each visit; and (10) addressing need for further consultations and how these consultations can be optimized.

How can this synthesis of alternative and mainstream treatment be achieved without burdening a dwindling pool of allergists with an additional fellowship in the middle or end of an established career? (By the way, they have plenty to keep them busy between the 40-yard lines of standard allergy care.)

Thus came Dr. Li's vision of a "Center for Integrative Medicine for Allergies and Wellness." The idea of integrative medicine is popular now. Memorial Sloan Kettering Cancer Center offers services to "complement mainstream cancer care (including) touch therapy, mind-body therapy, acupuncture, creative therapy, and nutrition counseling, as well as exercise programs to improve strength and promote relaxation." Many of these elements have analogues in TCM, and indeed, some of them are derived from it. The biggest

涉及 CAM 问题和/或疗效影响的医患互动的主要因素包括以下内容:(1)探索对 CAM 感兴趣的因素;(2)记录寻找 CAM 选项的临床原因;(3)评估迄今为止的疾病/健康状况和治疗方法;(4)记录患者的偏好和原因;(5)评估并记录医疗评估的充分性;(6)确定随访计划;(7)对于其他协商访问提供带有选项的良好风险沟通;(8)确认不断变化的期望和目标;(9)在每次拜访期间,对有关 CAM 选择的新的安全和/或疗效问题进行教育;(10)处理进一步咨询的需求以及如何优化这些咨询。

如何才能实现这种替代疗法和主流疗法的结合,而不让越来越少的过敏症专科医生在其职业生涯的中期或末期获得额外的奖金?(顺便说一句,在标准过敏治疗来回推翻、重建过程中,他们有很多事情要忙。)

由此李秀敏博士的愿景是"过敏和健康中西医结合中心"。中西医结合的想法现在很流行。纪念斯隆-凯特琳癌症中心提供的服务来"补充主流癌症护理(包括)触摸疗法、身心疗法、针灸疗法、创造性疗法、营养咨询以及提高力量和促进放松的锻炼计划。"这些元素中的很多在中医中具有类似物,而事实上,一些元素来源于中医。斯隆-凯特琳模

difference between the Sloan Kettering model and Dr. Li's vision is that hers carries with it a pharmacopeia to treat disease, not just to enhance patients' overall health while they endure chemotherapy and radiation.

Furthering the synthesis of TCM with Western medicine, which is called "translational research," Dr. Li's center will bridge the two worlds of medicine both for science and for treatment.

The parallel tracks of pioneering research and active current clinical practice give Dr. Li a unique advantage. For one thing, the fact that she works with therapies similar to those that are already available by prescription in China and Japan gives the medicines created under her supervision a leg up in the US approval process. Her private practice has grown without any Web presence or advertising. She started it because she wanted to provide an option for the families and patients who are interested in TCM but weren't qualified for or didn't want to take part in trials. She says,

In general, the patients and families find me though a referral from my colleagues at Mount Sinai, or other pediatricians, allergists, and dermatologists as well as the families. Family referral is becoming more common now. For example, after I see the first member of the family then other members start coming, too. Usually I see the children first and then the parents. This is because family history is important to allergy. In addition, some people find me though the publications from my group.

型和李秀敏博士的愿景之间最大的区别是她的模型包含治疗疾病的药典,而不仅仅是在化疗和放疗的同时提高病人的整体健康水平。

李秀敏博士的研究中心将进一步促进中西医结合,这被称为"转化研究",它将基于科学和治疗,在两个医学领域架起一座桥梁。

开创性研究的并行轨迹和积极的临床实践使李秀敏博士有了一个独特的优势。首先,她的治疗方法与中国和日本的处方类似,这一事实使她监管下生产的药物在美国审批过程中得到了支持。在没有网络沟通或广告的情况下,她的私人诊所已经发展壮大。她说自己之所以这么做,是因为她想为那些没有资格参加或不想参加临床试验却对中医感兴趣的家庭和病人提供一个选择。她还说,

总的来说,病人和家庭通过我在西奈山的同事、其他儿科医生、过敏科医生、皮肤病专家以及家人的推荐找到我。目前亲友推荐变得很普遍。例如,我治疗完第一个家庭成员之后,紧接着其他成员也会来。通常我先给孩子看病,然后是父母。这是因为家族史对过敏是重要的。另外,一些人通过我们小组发表的论文找到我。

The second reason that Dr. Li's unique circumstances offer an intermediate road to treatment is that her private clinic provides a real-world context for study, which is often lacking with allergy-related research. Asthma trials, for example, have been explicitly criticized for being optimized to study conditions using a more homogeneous study population than would be likely to take the medicine, and producing results that are far more favorable than those obtained in actual patient use.[1] Dr. Li's private practice can encompass patients with a greater variety of conditions and ages. (Whatever their variations, however, all patients are required to be tested for IgE, liver function, and other measures to ensure that their data can be incorporated into larger studies.)

Even before Dr. Li's new center gets off the ground, however, she and her colleagues have improvised several models for extending her ideas into mainstream treatment. For one thing, the medical school students at Mount Sinai established an integrative-medicine club. Medical students and interns are spending their summer in her labs, doing research and helping draft case report manuscripts based on unique cases. Likewise, clinical fellows are continually doing research in her lab.

Dr. Li has also begun a pilot program at the initiative of an asthma specialist in California who wrote to her because he has a number of patients who do not respond to inhaled corticosteroids or omalizumab. They have agreed that the California doctor will supply detailed histories and measurements

李秀敏博士独特的情况为治疗提供过渡途径的第二个原因是她的私人诊所为研究提供现实世界的背景,而与过敏相关的研究往往缺乏这种环境。例如,哮喘试验被明确批评为了优化研究条件,使用了同一地域的研究群体而不是愿意参与试验的志愿者,并产生了比实际患者使用时更有利的结果。李秀敏博士的私人实践可包含更多不同病情和不同年龄的患者。(然而,无论他们的变化是什么,要求检测所有患者的 IgE、肝功能和其他检测项目以确保他们的数据纳入更大规模的研究中。)

然而,就在李秀敏博士的新中心启动前,她和同事们已经即兴建立了几个将她的想法推广到主流治疗中的模型。一方面,西奈山医学院的学生建立了中西医结合医学俱乐部。医学生和实习生在她的实验室度过暑假,做研究并在独特案例基础上帮助起草病例报告手稿。同样地,临床研究员在她的实验室继续做研究。

李秀敏博士也开始了加利福尼亚哮喘专家倡议的试点项目,这位专家曾写信给李秀敏博士,因为他有一些对吸入型皮质类固醇激素或奥马珠单抗无反应的患者。他们同意加利福尼亚医生提供这些患者的详细

① Paul M O'Byrne. Asthma in the real world[J]. Journal of Allergy and Clinical Immunology, 2013, 132(1): 70-71.

for these patients and Dr. Li will provide the medications and the strategies for treatment, which will be delivered locally but supervised by her at a distance.

Another integrative approach sprang from treatment of a young man with a history of eczema, asthma, food allergies, and environmental allergies. His mother wanted to have his environmental allergies treated by her local allergist with SLIT, an alternative to allergy shots. To avoid the risk that SLIT allergens would aggravate his eczema and asthma, they chose to attack these conditions through use of TCM as well as treatment of his food allergies. The two doctors have developed a collaborative relationship, and the mother is pleased enough with the results for her son thus far to volunteer to help raise funds for the next phase of research using B-FAHF-2.

Still another approach for bridging alternative and mainstream practice is for Dr. Li to mentor mainstream practitioners as an extension of her private clinical practice. She has reached out to a select set of allergists in New York with a set of parameters of the patients she wants to treat collaboratively, basically the "worst of the worst" cases. She says, "These are people who have nowhere else to turn." A history of severe food allergy reactions or an additional symptom such as bad asthma is considered off limits for most clinical trials.

Dr. Li has outlined a set of specific parameters for these referrals. What they have in common are proven links to other conditions that are taking a discernible toll on the patients' quality of life. Improvement in

病史和各项指标,李秀敏博士将提供药物和治疗策略,这些方法将在当地进行,但由她远距离监督。

另一种中西医结合方法源自一位患有湿疹、哮喘、食物过敏和环境过敏的年轻人的治疗中。他母亲想让当地的过敏症专科医生用 SLIT 来治疗他的环境过敏,SLIT 是一种替代过敏注射的方法。为了避免 SLIT 过敏原加重其湿疹和哮喘的风险,他们选择通过使用中医治疗他的食物过敏来应对这些症状。两位医生已经形成一种合作关系,该母亲对她儿子的结果感到非常高兴,因此自愿为使用 B-FAHF-2 进行下一阶段的研究筹集基金。

还有另一种方法来连接替代医学和主流疗法,即李秀敏博士指导主流疗法医师作为她的私人临床实践的延伸。她已经联系了纽约的一组精挑细选的过敏症专科医师,并提供了一系列她想要合作治疗的病人的指标,基本上是"最糟糕的"病例。她说:"这些人无处可去。"严重的食物过敏反应病史或其他症状,例如严重哮喘,在大多数临床试验中被认为是禁忌的。

李秀敏博士为这些转诊患者描述了一些特定指标。他们的共同之处是与其他疾病的联系,这些疾病对患者的生活质量造成了明显的影响。

these conditions serves as a marker for improvement in the underlying allergies. The parameters are listed below. (If they sound familiar, it is because they echo the kinds of comorbid illnesses described, and successfully treated, in the previous chapter.)

1. *Recalcitrant eczema associated with food allergy, with total IgE greater than 2000 and elevated peanut-specific IgE.* The reasons for this parameter are several. First, patients with levels that high are out of bounds even for other new treatments, let alone conventional ones. Peanut allergy might respond to anti-IgE therapy (omalizumab, or Xolair), although it is not currently approved for that purpose, but in any case, it does not work well or is not recommended for someone with IgE levels above 2000.

Second, as already discussed, patients outgrow peanut allergies only 20% of the time and have the most to gain. Third, peanut-allergic children with intractable eczema have persistently high rates of peanut-specific IgE even when they conscientiously avoid the allergen.

2. *Frequent reactions associated with food allergy that severely compromise patients' quality of life.* As the case of Julie in the previous chapter shows, food-allergy reactions can take over the life of a previously highly functioning patient. The continuous threat of reaction can result in anxiety levels so high that it becomes impossible to distinguish between *actual* exposure to allergens and *perceived* exposure. Even in clinical trials, anxiety can run so high that it occasionally becomes necessary to administer epinephrine when the patient has received a placebo.

这些指标的改善是潜在过敏症状改善的标志。指标如下(如果它们听起来很熟悉,那是因为它们与前一篇中描述并成功治疗的共病性疾病相呼应):

1. 与食物过敏相关的顽固性湿疹,总 IgE 大于 2 000 并且升高的花生特异性 IgE。制定这个指标的原因如下:第一,这种高水平的患者甚至不能接受其他新的治疗方法,更不用说传统的治疗方法了。花生过敏可能对抗 IgE 疗法(奥马珠单抗或 Xolair)有反应,尽管目前尚未批准用于此目的,但是在任何情况下,它的效果并不好,且不推荐给 IgE 水平高于 2 000 以上的人。

第二,正如已经讨论过的,患者长大后只有20%的概率摆脱花生过敏症,绝大部分是患上过敏。第三,患有顽固性湿疹的花生过敏儿童即使在有意识避免过敏原时,花生特异性 IgE 的发生率仍然居高不下。

2. 与食物过敏相关的频繁反应严重损害患者的生活质量。如上一篇朱莉的病例所示,食物过敏反应可占据先前完全正常的患者的生活。反应的持续威胁可导致焦虑程度如此之高,以至于无法分辨真实接触到的过敏原和感知到的接触。即使在临床试验中,焦虑发生率如此之高,以至于当患者接受安慰剂时,有时也需要使用肾上腺素。在这些情况下,

In these cases, the holistic model of treatment characteristic of TCM serves several purposes simultaneously, gaining the patient's trust to minimize anxiety while treating both the underlying immune disorders and the symptoms. In mainstream treatment, the psychology is often treated separately.

3. *Symptomatic EoE*. This is a big one for many reasons. It is one of a number of so-called mixed-type mediated food disorders. Sixty percent of EoE patients also have positive serum IgE to foods, according to the 2010 NIAID food allergy guidelines.[①] EoE is a relatively new allergic disease. It was not even mentioned in my copy of the *Atlas of Allergic Diseases*, which was published in 2002—eosinophilic gastritis, yes, EoE no.[②] The standard treatment is that frustrating combination of avoidance and steroids.[③] Aaron's case in the previous chapter was typical:He had both IgE-mediated food allergies and EoE. He was a typical patient:young and male, and subject to delayed-onset long-lasting symptoms that frequently result in failure to thrive. EoE is an automatic disqualifier for OIT in clinical trials and OIT offered by private practitioners for a very good reason:Doses of the allergen will provoke unpleasant symptoms of another disease.

4. *Symptomatic asthma/allergic rhinitis that can be treated along with food allergies*. Day by day, asthma and allergic rhinitis make patients more miserable than

中医特色整体治疗模式可以同时达到多种目的,在治疗潜在的免疫疾病和症状的同时,获得患者的信任,将焦虑降至最低。在主流治疗中,心理治疗往往是分开进行的。

3. 症状性EoE。这是一个很大的问题,原因很多。它是许多所谓的混合型介导食物紊乱之一。根据《2010国家过敏与传染性疾病研究所食物过敏指南》,百分之六十的EoE患者对食物的血清IgE呈阳性。EoE是一种相对较新的过敏性疾病。我手上的2002年出版的《过敏性疾病图谱》中甚至都没有收录,嗜酸性粒细胞性食管炎,也就是EoE。标准的治疗方法是令人失望的忌口和类固醇组合。前面章节中亚伦的案例是典型的:他同时患有IgE介导食物过敏和EoE。他是典型的患者:年轻的男性,并受到延迟的长期症状的影响导致患者无法茁壮成长。在临床试验中,EoE是临床试验中OIT的自动不合格指标,而私人医生提供OIT的理由非常充分:过敏原的剂量会引发另一种疾病的令人不愉快的症状。

4. 症状性哮喘/过敏性鼻炎可与食物过敏一起治疗。日复一日,哮喘和过敏性鼻炎使患者比食物过敏

① NIAID-Sponsored Expert Panel. Guidelines for the diagnosis and management of food allergy in the United States:report of the NIAID-Sponsored Expert Panel[J]. Journal of Allergy and Clinical Immunology, 2010, 126(6):S1 - S58.

② Lieberman P L, Blaiss M S. Atlas of allergic diseases[M]. Berlin:Springer, 2002.

③ Matthew G, Seema S A, Jonathan M S, et al. The management of eosinophilic esophagitis[J]. Journal of Allergy and Clinical Immunology (In Practice), 2013, 1(4):332 - 340.

food allergies do, provided, of course, the food allergies are controlled through avoidance. The threat of food allergies is demoralizing; the realities of asthma and allergic rhinitis are depressing, distracting, and conspicuous. These other allergic diseases are so much as part of everyday life that improvement can provide a significant marker for measuring the progress of fixing the immune system overall. Nasal symptoms and breathing will improve as the IgE mechanism is modulated toward normal.

All the above conditions have both objective and subjective outcomes. Patients who perceive improvement in their quality of life will be most likely to persevere while waiting for the more abstract benefits of food-allergy therapy take hold. Collaboration with the primary allergists to add complementary therapy will reinforce compliance while also transferring knowledge of a new and hopeful approach to an intractable problem.

Missing from this list of priority patients are those whose food allergies are well controlled because they are disciplined in their avoidance and for whom the sole monitoring tool is allergen-specific IgE in the blood. As mentioned, IgE is a poor indicator for clinical allergy. Some patients with relatively low blood IgE levels can experience anaphylaxis from minor exposures, whereas others with much higher levels can eat a food safely. For patients who have food allergies but no co-morbid allergies that can stand in for measuring treatment progress, Dr. Li is working on a more direct route to safety.

更痛苦,当然,前提是食物过敏是通过忌口来控制的。食物过敏的威胁是令人泄气的,哮喘和过敏性鼻炎的实际情况令人沮丧、难以专注和与众不同。这些其他过敏疾病在日常生活中很常见,任何改善都是测量整个免疫系统的进展的一个重要标记。随着IgE机制向正常方向调整,鼻部症状和呼吸都会有所改善。

上述情况既有客观结果,也有主观结果。那些认为生活质量有所改善的病人最有可能一边坚持,一边等待免疫疗法更加精确的疗效稳定下来。与主要过敏症专家合作,增加补充疗法,将加强依从性,同时也让人知道(他们对)解决棘手问题的新的、充满希望的方法(的需求)。

这份优先患者名单中缺少的是那些食物过敏症得到很好控制的患者,因为他们在避免食物过敏方面很自律,对他们来说,唯一的监测工具是血液中的过敏原特异性IgE。如前所述,IgE是临床过敏的不良指标。具有相对较低IgE水平的一些患者可能会因轻微暴露而发生过敏反应,而具有较高水平的其他患者可以安全饮食。患有食物过敏而无其他过敏症状的患者可参与检测治疗进程,李秀敏博士正在开发一种更直接的安全路径。

She says, we have identified several compounds from FAHF-2 and ASHMI that directly suppress IgE. Beyond FAHF-2 and ASHMI, we have built up an inventory of more than 1,000 TCMs at our lab. We used IgE-producing B-cell lines to screen the medicines with most potent IgE inhibitory effects and identify the active compounds. We have found two compounds that were very potent and safe in direct suppression of B-cell IgE production. My goal is a more potent and convenient natural treatment that reduces IgE quickly while still being very safe.

It must also be pointed out that for the time being, patients who visit the clinic will have to be sufficiently well off to afford these treatments, although the treatments are comparable in price to the OIT that many families are paying for out of pocket and to the combination of health care cost and income loss incurred by parents' sacrifice to help manage food allergies (chapter 1).

The parameters have now been shared with a select number of New York allergists, spearheaded by my cousin, Dr. Paul Ehrlich, who is perennially one of the top pediatric allergists in New York and past president of the New York Allergy and Asthma Society. Patients will be treated both by their own allergists and Dr. Li, and in the process, some of her approach will be shared with the mainstream doctors.

Dr. Li doesn't expect the mainstream physicians to become TCM doctors. "Younger physicians will be able to go further," she says. "Allergists who are just entering practice will have more time and incentive to learn."

她说：我们已经从 FAHF-2 和 ASHMI 中鉴定出几种直接抑制 IgE 的化合物。除了 FAHF-2 和 ASHMI，我们在实验室已经建立了一个超过 1 000 种中药的目录。我们使用产生 IgE 的 B 细胞株以筛选具有最强的 IgE 抑制效果的药物，并确定活性化合物。我们发现了在直接抑制 B 细胞 IgE 产生的非常有效和安全的两种化合物。我的目标是保证安全性的同时，找到一个更有效和更方便的快速减少 IgE 的自然疗法。

还必须指出的是，在目前的情况下，就诊的病人必须有足够的钱来支付这些治疗，尽管这种疗法的价格与许多家庭自掏腰包支付的 OIT 相当，也与父母为帮助应对食物过敏牺牲时间造成的收入损失和医疗费用相当（第 1 篇）。

这些指标目前与精挑细选的一些纽约过敏症专科医师共享，我的堂兄，保罗·埃尔利希博士，纽约顶尖儿科过敏症专科医师之一，并且是纽约过敏和哮喘协会的前任会长。李秀敏博士将和患者的过敏症专科医师共同治疗，并且她的方法将在治疗过程中和主流医生分享。

李秀敏博士不期望主流医生变成中医医生。她说："年轻的医生将走得更远，而刚开始执业的过敏症专科医师将有更多的时间和动力学习。"

One element that should be part of this collaboration is that each time a patient is referred to Dr. Li, the referring doctor should be present for the initial history, which takes up to two hours, not as a participant but as an observer. Dr. Li has told me that it is her goal, and a goal of Chinese medicine, to treat the whole person. She seeks in this first consultation to try to get a sense of not only the extent of the disease but also the underlying pathology that may be contributing to the disease's severity before she concludes whether she can help someone. This is a two-way street—the patient must also have confidence in her. Such individuation may take the direction of the first meeting down several paths. It may lead in some instances to an acupuncture treatment, as in the case of Julie, whose very real experience of repeated anaphylaxis had led to extreme anxiety. (Acupuncture, as mentioned above, is one of the few alternative treatments that has earned limited approval by NCCAM and is reimbursable by many health insurance companies.) Or the initial visit may be all talk and examination.

Enthralled though I am with Dr. Li's approach, I recognize that this kindly doctor, time-is-no-object history isn't something that only TCM practitioners do. I have watched my cousin take long histories from new patients (with their permission for me to observe), and I have seen the part it can play in gaining patient confidence as well as gaining valuable clues to patient allergies. In Dr. Groopman's book *How Doctors Think*, he recounts several cases in which patients have been studied and treated unsuccessfully for months or years and have achieved a breakthrough only when a new and wise doctor ignores reams of charts and tests and

这种合作的一个组成部分是每次向李秀敏博士推荐患者,介绍初始病史的两个多小时内推荐医师应在场,不是作为参与者而是作为观察者。李医生告诉我,整体治疗是她的目标,也是中医的目标。在她断定是否能帮助某人之前,她在首次咨询中试图了解疾病程度和可能导致疾病的严重程度的潜在病理。这个过程是双向的,患者也必须对她有信心。这种个性化可能将首次见面的方向转向几个路径。在某些情况下,可能采用针灸治疗,如朱莉病例中所述,朱莉反复出现过敏反应的真实经历导致了极度的焦虑。(如上所述,针灸疗法是为数不多的通过 NCCAM 批准的有限的替代疗法之一,并且在许多医疗保险公司是可以报销的。)或者,首次交流可能全部都是谈话和检查。

尽管我被李秀敏博士的方法迷住,但是我意识到这位和蔼的医生所说的"治疗时间不是目的"并不是只有中医执业医师能做的事。我看到我的堂兄花费很长的时间治疗新患者(他们允许我进行观察),并且我看到了它在建立病人信心以及获得病人过敏的宝贵线索方面所起的作用。在讲述古罗柏曼医师想法的书《医生如何思考》中,他叙述了几个案例,在这些案例中,医生在研究和治疗病人上花费了数月甚至数年,但只有当一个新的、明智的医生忽略大

asks the patient to begin at the beginning. Groopman and Dr. Lisa Sanders place great stock in the importance of narrative and feeling in diagnosis.

Although healers of various scientific traditions may have many things in common, there are differences among them and strengths in each. Dr. Li says, "Western medicine is great in some areas such as surgery and infectious diseases, and TCM is great in others." The instance of EoE is a case in point of the limitations of the Western approach. Avoidance is a sensible strategy as far as it goes, and so is the use of steroids for flares, but EoE and probably all other food allergies are digestive diseases as well as immune disorders, and so the TCM approach is to treat the digestive tract as well as practicing avoidance and immune suppression. TCM practitioners look at eczema and see several possible diseases involving different parts of the body. Treating the skin with steroids while avoiding allergenic triggers only goes so far. Jackie's history (see previous chapter) reads like a kind of guide to the medical schools of the Ivy League. These doctors, like my cousin, did their best, but the patient didn't get better until he worked with Dr. Li.

Dr. Li comes to these initial meetings prepared not only to take a long history and to gain the confidence of both patient and parents, but also with a command of what amounts to an entirely new set of tools for treatment, although of course they are not new to her. This is the original holistic medicine.

To conclude, I turn again to Dr. Engler, who told me: "We have lost connection with patient

量的图表和测试,并要求病人从头开始时,他们才取得了突破。曼和丽莎·桑德斯博士非常重视叙述的重要性和诊断中的感受。

尽管不同科学传统的治疗师可能有许多共同之处,但他们各有不同之处,且各有所长。李秀敏博士说:"西医在一些领域如外科手术和传染病等方面效果很好,而中医在其他方面效果也很好。"EoE 的例子是西医方法局限性的最佳体现。就现状来说,忌口是明智的策略,使用类固醇治疗过敏症状加重也是如此,但是EoE 和其他所有食物过敏属于消化性疾病以及免疫功能紊乱,因此,中医方法用于治疗消化系统(疾病)以及实施忌口和免疫抑制。中医师观察湿疹,可能发现几种涉及身体不同部位的疾病。用类固醇治疗皮肤,同时避免过敏性触发物只能到此为止。杰基的病史(见前面章节)读起来像常春藤盟校医学院的指南。这些医生,比如我的堂兄,尽了自己最大的努力,但是直到与李秀敏博士合作,患者的情况才好转。

李秀敏博士想起拟定的初始会面,不仅要花很长时间获得患者和父母的信心,还要掌握一套全新的治疗手段。当然,尽管对她来说并不新颖。这就是原始的整体医学。

总而言之,我再一次回顾恩格勒博士对我说的话:"我们与患者的故

stories. Patients who don't fit are marginalized. Doctors should expand their medical toolbox for patients who don't fall within guidelines. We need a mechanism for compassionate trials. Dr. Li's work is a flag in the desert. It's beautiful science. "

事失去了联系。不符合条件的患者被边缘化。医生应该为不符合指导方针的病人扩大他们的医疗手段。我们需要富有同情心的试验机制。李秀敏博士的工作是沙漠里的一面旗帜。科学是美丽的。"

Appendix

What It Is Like to Participate in a FAHF-2 Clinical Trial—One Mother's Account

（Note—this account is for information about the process and its effects on a participant. The results of this trial have not yet been published.）

The FAHF-2 clinical trials are blind and anonymous from the medical side; however, there's nothing to stop participants and their families from discussing their experience, and with the instant publication opportunities afforded by the Internet, their thoughts can find a worldwide audience. One mother writing as Food Allergy Bitch（FAB）has chronicled her son's participation in a FAHF-2 trial. I reached out to her through her Twitter account, and she wrote back to me through an anonymous e-mail account.

FAB's son—I'll call him Sam—was allergic to cow's milk, soy, peanuts, and most peas and beans. FAB kept current with research through a support board she ran online, dismissing OIT trials because "we had heard from people participating how difficult it was to keep the allergen in the diet each day and how tolerances could just suddenly shift, resulting in serious reactions." When allergist Dr. Sakina Bajowala wrote favorably about FAHF-2 in her blog, The Allergist

附 录

参与 FAHF-2 临床试验是什么感觉——一个母亲的描述

（注：该描述是关于治疗过程的信息以及对参与者的影响。本次试验的结果还未发布。）

FAHF-2 临床试验从医学角度来说是盲目的和匿名的。然而，没有什么事情可阻止参与者和其家庭讨论他们的经历，并且随着互联网提供的即时发布机会，他们的想法会得到全世界的关注。一位母亲以"食物过敏这件麻烦事（FAB）"的身份记录了她的儿子参与 FAHF-2 试验。我试图通过她的推特账号与她沟通，她通过匿名电子邮件账户回复我。

"FAB"的儿子——我称他为萨姆——对牛奶、大豆、花生和大多数豌豆和豆类过敏。"FAB"通过她在网上运营的一个支持委员会不断了解最新的研究，控诉 OIT 试验，因为"我们从参与的人们那里听说，每天对饮食中那么多东西过敏是多么困难，以及耐受性是如何突然转变的，从而导致严重的反应。"当过敏症专科

Mommy,[①] FAB decided to apply. A complete two-day examination included spirometry, a cardiac assessment, blood work, and SPT. The crux of the screening was a placebo-controlled peanut challenge—ground peanut disguised by applesauce or plain applesauce for the placebo—to find out if he was truly peanut allergic. His threshold for peanut going in was high enough that, unlike for many other peanut-allergic patients, cross-contamination was not considered a mortal threat.

FAB writes, "They were very cautious with my son because he tends to have slow-building reactions—it took a full 15 minutes on the SPT before his wheal showed up. They left a lot of time between doses to make sure everything wouldn't suddenly hit him." Despite low IgE numbers and moderate skin reactions to peanut during the screening, the young man exhibited escalating reactions as larger doses were given, and the challenge was terminated at a level of three peanuts. (A complete and vivid account of this experience is available on FAB's blog.[②])

Responding to my questions, FAB describes her son's state of mind as the trial began: "He didn't have a lot of hope about it. I think one surprising thing I've learned from all of this is that he's made his peace with the life he has to lead. He expects to be allergic to cow's milk the rest of his life, which severely limits his ability to eat out. He did the trial because he really

医师萨吉娜·巴窝瓦拉博士在她的博客中写到 FAHF-2 的有利的一面时,过敏患者的母亲"FAB"决定采纳。整整两天的检查包括肺活量测定、心脏评估、血液检查和皮肤点刺试验。筛选的关键是安慰剂对照花生诱导——用苹果酱伪造成花生碎或纯苹果酱作为安慰剂——以确定他是否真是花生过敏。与所有其他花生过敏患者不同,他摄入花生的阈值足够高,交叉感染不被视为致命的威胁。

"FAB"写道:"他们非常谨慎地对待我的儿子,因为他反应迟缓——在他出现水疱之前,在皮肤点刺试验中消耗了整整 15 分钟的时间。注射剂量间隔很长,以确保他不会突然产生反应。"尽管在筛查过程中 IgE 值较低,皮肤对花生的反应也较为温和,但随着剂量的增加,这名年轻男子的反应却在不断升级,最终在 3 颗花生的水平上结束了挑战。("FAB"的博客上有关于这次经历的完整而生动的描述。)

在回答我的问题时,"FAB"描述了她的儿子随着试验开始后的心理状态:"他对此没有抱太大的希望。我认为我从这些当中学到的一件令人惊奇的事是他已经平静地接受了他必须过的生活。他预计余生都会对牛奶过敏,将严重限制他外出吃饭。他做试验是因为他真的相信自己是

---

① http://allergistmommy. blogspot. eom/2010/09/chinese-herbal-for- mula-to-protect. html.

② http://foodallergybitch. blogspot. com/2012/04/btdt-got-fahf-2-food-allergy-clinical. html.

believed he was helping science, not because he expected a miracle cure. " For herself: "My fears were the obvious ones: I knew he was going to have to go through at least three reactions. The doctors assured us over and over again that there would be as little danger as possible, but of course you're always thinking about the one-in-a-million chance when you're a mom. The other fear was that my son would resent me for putting him through all of it. I do feel like I was the one pushing. "

As discussed, compliance presented a series of challenges: Ten pills slightly bigger than M&M's three times a day, ideally at least four hours apart and with meals. "He was a typical teenager and we started this trial in April, so much of the medication dosing happened over the summer. That could mean his last meal was 6:00 with the family, or at 11:00 at night depending on his work and social schedule. " His high school was very strict. "We needed a letter from the trial and he had to take his lunch dose in the nurse's office each day. She was really great about it all, though, and really interested in the trial itself, as there are many other kids in the school with allergies. "

Each dose was documented for the study in a log, and when he spent a week at camp, FAB tore a week of the log out and sent it, along with his pills, with him. The camp was much more relaxed about his regimen than the high school.

For six months, taking 30 pills a day, Sam kept a journal as part of the trial, but he really didn't notice any notable side effects, gastric or otherwise. After six

在帮助科学,而不是因为他期待奇迹般的治愈,所以他进行了试验。"对于"FAB"自己而言:"我的恐惧是明显的,我知道他将经历至少三个反应。医生一再地向我们保证会尽可能地将危险降低。但是,当然,当你作为一位母亲时,你总会想到百万分之一的概率。另一个担心是,我儿子会因为我让他经历了这一切而怨恨我。我确实感觉是我在推动这件事。"

如先前所讨论的,依从性带来了一系列的挑战:10 片略大于 M&M's 巧克力豆的药丸,一天三次,理想情况下至少间隔四个小时,并在用餐时服用。"他是典型青少年,我们在四月份开始了这个试验,整个夏天要服用这么多的药物剂量。这可能意味着他和家人的最后一顿饭是早上6:00或晚上 11:00,这取决于他的工作和社交安排。"他的高中非常严格。"我们需要一封试验信函,而且,他每天必须在护士办公室服用他的午餐剂量。但是,护士真的做得很棒,她真的对试验本身很感兴趣。因为学校里还有很多其他患有过敏症的孩子。"

试验的每次剂量都记录在日志中,当他要在露营地度过一周时,"FAB"将一周的日志撕下,并连同他的药丸一起给他。露营地对他的服药方案执行比高中宽松。

六个月,每天服用 30 片药丸,作为试验的一部分,萨姆坚持写日记。但是他确实没有注意到任何明显的副作用,无论是胃还是其他方面。六

months were up, he returned for the same round of applesauce with peanut powder. This time, he was able to eat the equivalent of nine peanuts.

Three months after Sam stopped taking the medication, he returned to see if the gains had been maintained. "They had," FAB reports. "He got to the dose just below the dose he achieved in October. He might have been able to push to one more, but there's an art to making sure these kids don't tip over into a serious reaction, and the researchers are cautious about not exceeding that magic window."

For this family, however, peanuts were not the crucial allergen. Would the protection extend to his big one—milk? Prior to the trial, Sam underwent a challenge and was able to tolerate milk in some forms: small amounts of baked milk, but not baked cheese, with some oral reactions during the challenge. All forms of milk were avoided during therapy, but afterward, food with baked milk and butter were introduced to his diet without incident.

Another big allergen for Sam was soy, which had resulted in an epinephrine injection and a trip to the ER during his freshman year in high school. "In February, we took him in for a soy challenge at his regular allergist. He passed! He has successfully added soy back into his diet at this point, although again, we're proceeding cautiously. However, he's eating Ramen noodles almost daily and has added a number of processed Chinese foods."

FAB says, "My overall assessment of participating is positive … and wishy-washy." While she believes they have seen real benefits from the medication, she

个月结束以后,他又进行一轮含有花生粉的苹果酱试验。这一次,他能够食用的食物等量于9个花生。

萨姆停止服药后三个月内,又回来看这种效果是否能保持住。"FAB"报道:"效果保持住了。他的服药剂量低于十月份的。他也许能够再上一层楼,但是必须有确保这些孩子不陷入严重反应的技术,并且研究人员对不超出这个令人惊讶的效果持谨慎态度。"

然而,对于这个家庭而言,花生不是主要的过敏原。这种保护能延伸到他的更严重的过敏原牛奶吗?在试验之前,萨姆接受了刺激并能够忍受一些形式的牛奶:微量的烘焙牛奶而不是烘焙奶酪,在刺激期间具有一些口腔反应。在治疗期间,应避免食用任何形式的牛奶,但之后,他的饮食中加入了烘焙牛奶和黄油,没有发生任何意外。

萨姆的另一大过敏原是大豆,这导致他曾在高中一年级注射肾上腺素并被送去急诊室。"我们带他去他的常规过敏专科医生那里参加了一次大豆挑战。他通过了!他已经成功地将大豆添加到他的饮食中,尽管我们谨慎地进行着。然而,他几乎每天都吃日本拉面,并添加了一些中国加工食品。"

"FAB"说:"我对参与的总体评价是积极的但浅显的。"虽然她相信受试者已经看到了药物治疗的真正

acknowledges that those benefits may not extend to all patients. "The study results are due out soon, and hopefully we'll know then whether this treatment will be appropriate for all individuals with food allergies. There are no firm answers at the end. The work that's being done is for the benefit of science and any benefit to your child is almost incidental. You don't know if it will work, or how it works. We do not have any specific instructions about how to proceed now that the trial is done. We are all waiting to see, once the results are published, if it was a success. "

好处,但她认为,这些好处可能不会惠及所有患者。"研究结果很快就要发布了,希望届时我们会知道这个治疗方法是否适用于所有食物过敏的人。最终不会有固定答案。正在做的工作是为了科学,而对你的孩子的任何好处几乎都是偶然的。你不知道它是否生效,或如何生效。现在试验已经完成,我们没有接到任何具体的指示接下来如何进行。我们都在等待结果发布,看它是否成功。"

ACKNOWLEDGMENTS

First, I must thank Dr. Xiu-Min Li of Mount Sinai School of Medicine for entrusting me with the privilege of telling the story of her work. I can't say enough about her and my esteem for her, but in the pages that follow, you will get the picture. I would also like to thank my co-authors Dr. Larry Chiaramonte and Dr. Paul Ehrlich for making me their collaborator over a long time, and imparting to me their inquisitive and patient-centered approach to medicine.

Next, Linda J. Miller, PhD; Arnold I. Levinson, MD; Anne F. Russell BSN, RN, AE-C; Jessica Martin, PhD; Mark Cullen, MD; and Adolph Singer, MD for reading the manuscript at various stages and offering suggestions, particularly on the credibility of the science, and its presentation.

Thanks, also, to Hugh Sampson, MD, who heads the Jaffe Food Allergy Institute at Mount Sinai, and his colleagues at Sinai Scott Sicherer, MD; Julie Wang, MD; Anna Nowak Wegzryn, MD; and Ying Song, MD, for talking to me about various aspects of the work. And to David Dunkin, MD and Jessica Reid-Adam, MD for discussing their very exciting research.

致　谢

首先,我必须感谢西奈山医学院的李秀敏博士对我的信任,授权给我讲述有关她工作的故事。对于她,我怎样褒奖也不为过,对她的尊重我也是无法用语言表达的,但你可以在接下来的篇章中感受到。我也要感谢我的合著者们——拉里·基亚拉蒙特博士和保罗·埃尔利希博士。感谢他们愿意与我长期合作,并且把他们追根究底和以病人为中心的医学理念传授给我。

其次,感谢琳达·J.米勒(博士),阿诺德·I.莱文森(医学博士),安妮·F.拉塞尔(护理学士,注册护士),杰西卡·马丁(博士),马克·卡伦(医学博士)和阿道夫·辛格(医学博士),他们在写作的不同阶段阅读手稿并且给我提出建议,特别是在研究的科学可信度以及描述方面。

同样要感谢西奈山贾菲食品过敏研究所的会长休·桑普森医学博士和他在西奈山的同事们——斯科特·史可瑞医学博士、朱莉·王医学博士、安娜·诺瓦卡·威格森医学博士和宋颖医学博士,是他们告诉我有关于这项工作的方方面面。我还要感谢大卫·邓金医学博士和杰西卡·里德·亚当医学博士跟我讨论了他们非常振奋人心的研究。

179

Dr. Renata Engler, has been especially helpful for her long-time appreciation in print and in person of Dr. Li's work, her incisive critique of the shortcomings of Western medicine in treating allergic disease, her framework for the possible incorporation of complementary and alternative medicine in American clinical practice, and for her spontaneous eloquence.

Thanks also to my old friend Tim Koranda for answering questions about Chinese culture.

Finally, I have enjoyed the support and advice of Susan Weissman, author of *Feeding Eden: the Trials and Triumphs of a Food Allergy Family*, the best memoir of negotiating the challenges of this epidemic I can imagine.

勒娜特·恩格勒博士也给我提供了帮助,尤其感谢长期以来她在本书印刷中所做的贡献,感谢她在李秀敏博士工作中对西方医学治疗过敏疾病的缺点的深刻评论和她提出的在美国临床实践中纳入补充替代医学的构思,以及她天生的好口才。

同时感谢我的老朋友蒂姆·科兰达回答我关于中国文化的问题。

最后,我也得到了《喂养伊顿:一个食物过敏家庭的试验和胜利》一书的作者苏珊·韦思曼的支持和建议,该书是我所能想到的关于成功挑战食物过敏这一流行病的最好的回忆录。